DR. SEBI

BOOK OF OF REMEDIES

Alkaline Medicine Making and Herbal Remedies for Common Ailments | Boost Immunity, Improve Health and Life-Long Vitality

---

BY

KERRI M. WILLIAMS

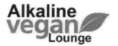

www.alkalineveganlounge.com

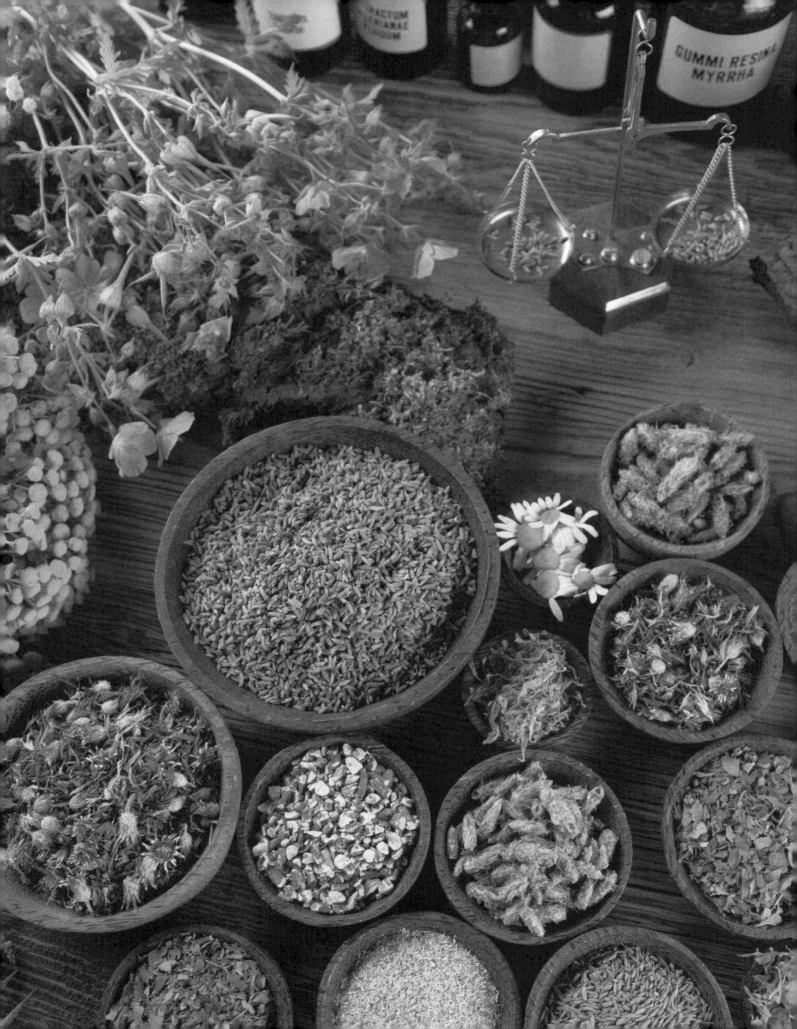

CONTENTS

INTRODUCTION — XIII
THE AWAKENING — XVI

CHAPTER 1: — 1

THE DR. SEBI ALKALINE DIET — 1
DR. SEBI ELECTRIC DIET VS CONVENTIONAL ALKALINE DIET — 2

DR. SEBI REMEDIES AND RECIPES — 3

ABSCESS AND GINGIVITIS — 3
REMEDIES — 3
HERBAL MOUTHWASH — 3
SKIN ABSCESS FIGHTING TEA — 4
TOPICAL WASH FOR ABSCESSES AND GINGIVITIS — 5

ACNE — 7
REMEDIES — 7
SKIN TONER — 7
FACIAL STEAM — 8
ACNE-FIGHTING TEA — 9
ACNE WASH — 9

AGING — 11
REMEDIES — 11
ANTI-AGING TEA 1 — 11
ANTI-AGING TEA 2 — 11

ALLERGIES — 13
REMEDIES — 13
ALLERGY RELIEF TEA — 13
QUICK ALLERGY TEA — 13
FLOWER DECOCTION — 14
NETTLE TEA — 15

ANEMIA — 16
REMEDIES — 16
Anemia Tea — 16

ARTHRITIS — 17
REMEDIES — 17
Arthritis Milding Tea — 17
Quick Analgesic Arthritis Tea — 17
Nightly Arthritis Tea — 18
Arthritis Ointment — 19

ASTHMA — 21
REMEDIES — 21
Quick Acting Asthma Tea — 21
Soothing Tea — 22

AUTISM — 23
REMEDIES — 23
Autistic Treatment — 23
Dietary Changes — 23

BACK PAIN — 24
REMEDIES — 24
Spine's Fine Tincture — 24
Warming Compress — 24
Sciatic Pain Tea — 24
Analgesic Daily Tea for Back Pain — 25
Soothing Back Pain Tea — 25

BEDSORES — 26
REMEDIES — 26
Bedsore Topical Wash — 26
But Bite Relief Spray — 27
Topical Wash for Bites and Stings — 27
Skin Soothing Ointment — 27

BRONCHITIS — 29
REMEDIES — 29
Fire Cider — 29
Throat Soothing tea — 29
Sweet Soothing Tea — 29

BURNS AND SUNBURNS — 31
REMEDIES — 31
BURN HEALING HONEY — 31
SUNBURN SPRAY — 31
BURN POULTICE — 31
IMMUNITY STRENGTHENER — 31

COLD SORES — 33
REMEDIES — 33
COLD SORE COMPRESS — 33
COLD SORE BALM — 33
COLD SORE TEA — 33
COLD SORE MOUTHWASH — 34

CONSTIPATION — 35
REMEDIES — 35
BOWEL-HYDRATING INFUSION — 35
BOWEL-MOTIVATING TINCTURE — 35
BOWEL-SOOTHING TEA — 35
PURIFYING DIGESTIVE TEA — 36

COUGH AND COLD — 37
REMEDIES — 37
LUNG LUBRICATING TEA — 37
ANTITUSSIVE OXYMEL — 37
COUGH SYRUP — 37
SOOTHING COUGH AND COLD FORMULA — 38
LAKOTA COUGH AND COLD FORMULA — 38
LUMBEE COUGH AND COLD FORMULA — 39
QUICK ACTING COUGH AND COLD FORMULA — 39
EXPECTORATING COUGH AND COLD TEA — 40
DECONGESTANT TEA — 40
ANTITUSSIVE FLOWER TEA — 40
QUICK-ACTING MULLEIN COUGH SYRUP — 41
ELECAMPANE COUGH SYRUP — 41
HOREHOUND LOZENGES — 41

CRAMPS — 43
REMEDIES — 43
MUSCLE WARMING OINTMENT — 43
MUSCLE CRAMP TEA — 43

MUSCLE RUB	43
DIARRHEA	**45**
REMEDIES	**45**
ASTRINGENT TEA	45
CINNAMON POWDER CAPSULES	45
QUICK AND EASY DIARRHEA TEA	46
SOOTHING DIARRHEA TEA	46
IROQUOIS TEA	46
FATIGUE	**47**
REMEDIES	**47**
SHAKE-IT-OFF FORMULA	47
UP AND ABOUT MORSELS	47
PICK-ME-UP TEA	48
INVIGORATING TEA	48
FEVER	**49**
REMEDIES	**49**
FEVER-REDUCING TEA	49
FEVER-BREAKING TEA	49
QUICK-ACTING FEVER TEA	50
FOOD INTOLERANCES	**51**
REMEDIES	**51**
GUT-HEAL TEA	51
BUILD-UP BROTH	51
STOP FLATULENCE TEA	52
COLON-SOOTHING TEA	52
QUICK-ACTING FLATULENCE TEA	52
GUT-CLEARING TEA	52
DAILY DIGESTIVE TEA	53
PEPPERY INDIGESTION TEA	53
HANGOVER	**55**
REMEDIES	**55**
TAKE-IT-EASY NEXT DAY INFUSION	55
NO-FUSS HANGOVER TEA	55
QUICK-ACTING HANGOVER TEA	55
SPICY HANGOVER TEA	56

HEADACHE — 57
REMEDIES — 57
COOLING HEADACHE TEA — 57
WARMING HEADACHE TEA — 57
PEPPERY HEADACHE TEA — 57
SOOTHING HEADACHE TEA — 58

HEARTBURN/REFLUX/GERD — 59
REMEDIES — 59
MARSHMALLOW INFUSION — 59
PREVENTATIVE BITTER TINCTURE — 59
QUICK-ACTING HEARTBURN TEA — 59
SOOTHING HEARTBURN TEA — 60

INDIGESTION/DYSPEPSIA — 61
REMEDIES — 61
PRE-EMPTIVE BITTER TINCTURE — 61
CARMINATIVE TINCTURE — 61
DIGESTIVE TEA — 61
STRONG DIGESTIVE TEA — 62
QUICK-ACTING DIGESTIVE TEA — 62

INSOMNIA — 63
REMEDIES — 63
END-OF-THE-DAY ELIXIR — 63
SLEEP FORMULA — 63
INSOMNIA RELIEF TEA — 64
SWEET DREAMS TEA — 64

MENSTRUAL CYCLE IRREGULARITIES — 65
REMEDIES — 65
STEADY CYCLE TEA — 65
BLEED ON TEA — 66
DAILY SOOTHING MENSTRUAL TEA — 66
DYSMENORRHEA TEA — 66
CRAMP RELIEF TEA — 67

NAUSEA AND VOMITING — 67
REMEDIES — 67
CALMING TEA — 67

RASH — 69
REMEDIES — 69
- Weepy Rash Poultice — 69
- Skin-Soothing Tea — 70
- Rash Wash — 70

SINUSITIS/STUFFY NOSE — 71
REMEDIES — 71
- Sinus-Clearing Steam Bath — 71
- Sinus-Relieving Tea — 71
- Mucous-Freeing Tea — 71

SORE THROAT — 72
REMEDIES — 72
- Sore Throat Tea — 72
- Herbal Gargle — 72
- Throat-Soothing Tea — 73
- Fruity Gargle — 73
- Sweet Cough Drops — 74

SPRAINS AND STRAINS — 75
REMEDIES — 75
- Soft Tissue Injury Liniment — 75
- Topical Pain Relief — 75
- Quick-Acting Pain Relief — 76
- Sweet Relief Tea — 76

STRESS — 77
REMEDIES — 77
- Rescue Elixir — 77
- Soothe Up Tea — 77
- Nerve Soothing Tea — 77
- Calming Tea — 77
- Shake-It-Off Tea — 78

WEIGHT LOSS AND BELLY FAT — 79
REMEDIES — 79

WOUNDS — 79
REMEDIES — 79
- Wound Wash — 79

Pine Resin Salve — 79
Topical Application for Abrasions — 80
Topical Wash for Cuts — 80

BONUS RECIPES — 83

1. Roasted Okra with Habanero — 83
2. Roasted Okra with Tomatoes — 83
3. Mushrooms Stuffed Avocados — 84
4. Roasted Okra with Lime and Dill — 85
5. Avocado and Squash — 85
6. Okra with Onion and Tomato — 86
7. Avocado Lettuce Wrap — 87
8. Pepper and Lettuce Wrap — 87
9. Squash with Sage — 88
10. Peppers Stuffed Mushrooms — 89
11. Tomato and Onion Stuffed Zucchini — 90
12. Mushrooms Stuffed with Onion and Tomatoes — 90
13. Zucchini Noodles with Tomatoes — 91
14. Okra Lettuce Wrap — 92
15. Bell Pepper Stuffed with Wild Rice — 93
16. Wild Rice with Chickpeas and Mushrooms — 93
17. Wild Rice with Bell Peppers and Turnip Greens — 94
18. Wild Rice and Tomato Lettuce Wrap — 95
19. Bell Pepper Stuffed Tef — 95
20. Wild Rice Stuffed Mushrooms — Error! Bookmark not defined.
21. Chickpeas and Olives with Wild Rice — Error! Bookmark not defined.
22. Wild Rice with Chickpeas, Squash and kale — Error! Bookmark not defined.
23. Wild Rice with Chickpeas and Red Bell Pepper — Error! Bookmark not defined.
24. Okra with Wild Rice — Error! Bookmark not defined.
25. Mushrooms Stuffed with Quinoa — Error! Bookmark not defined.

RELATED BOOK YOU MAY LIKE — 97

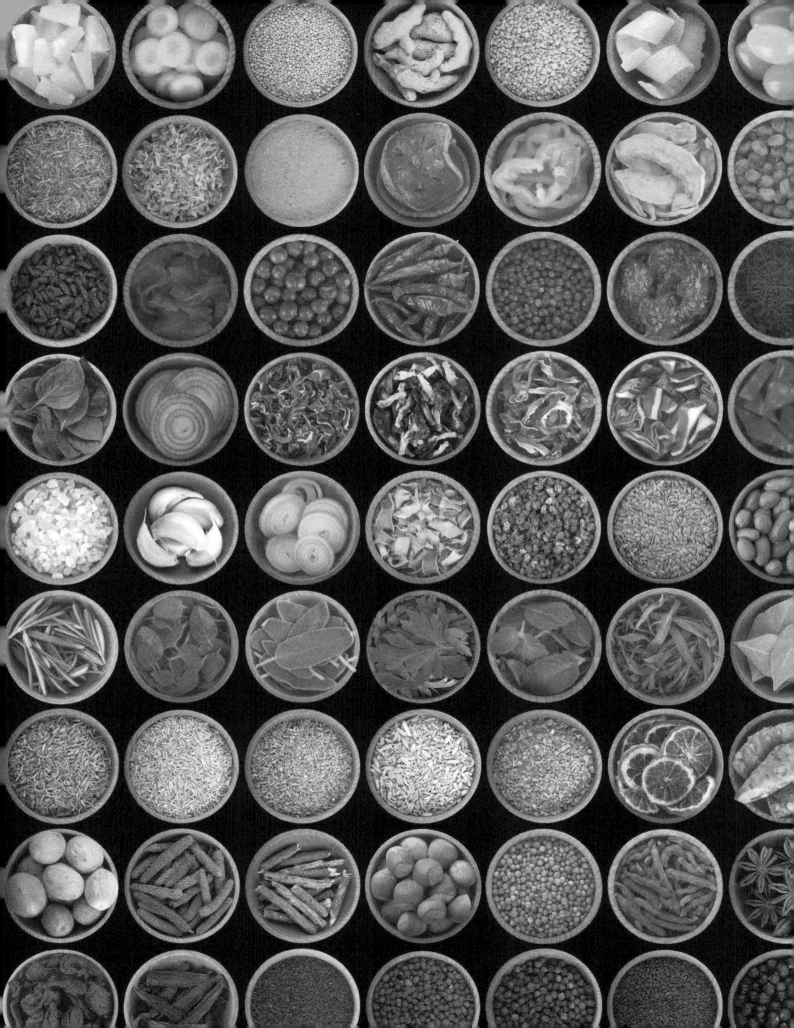

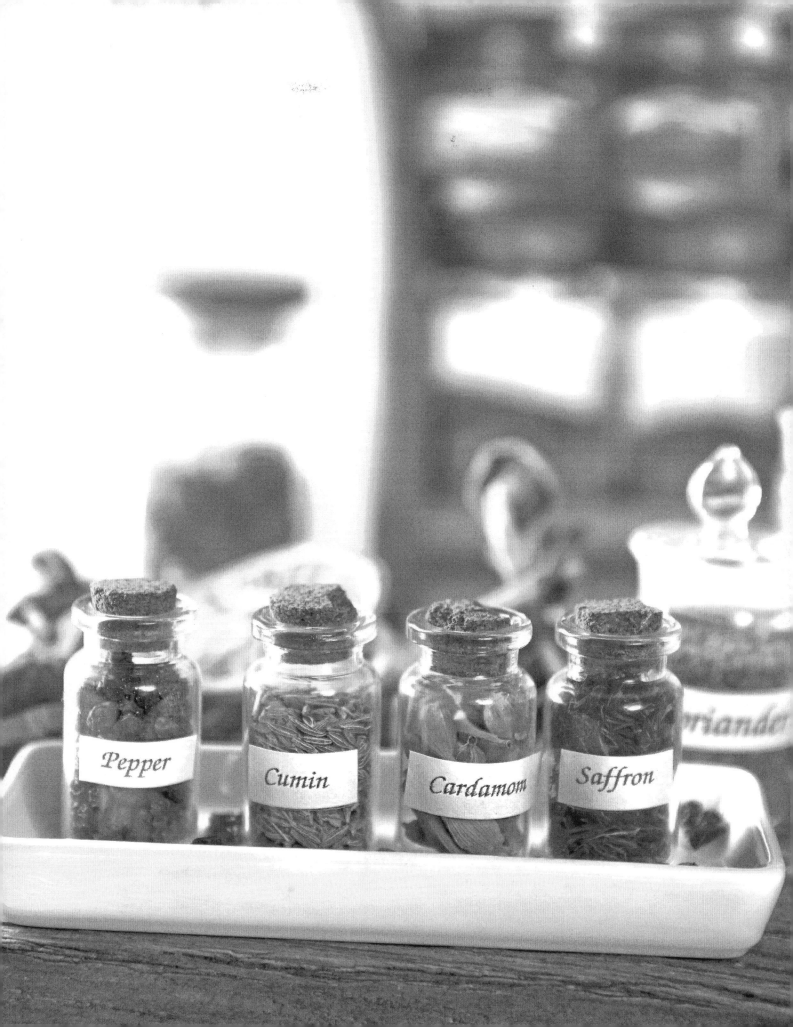

DEDICATION

To the only one healer who spoke the truth, preached the truth and lived and died for the truth. Rest in Power, Dr. Sebi.

JOIN OUR COMMUNITY

Join our community of growing enthusiasts committed to the lifestyle. Also, we occasionally run discount promos for our books and other resources, and you'd be pleased to sign up to our exclusive list to get access for free. It's an amazing and growing community where we share tips and resources to help in our journey towards healthy living. Copy the link below and paste into your browser to join for free

https://manage.kmail-lists.com/subscriptions/subscribe?a=X7eqXQ&g=YdcvB2

FREE SEBI DIET STARTER KIT

Download our free Dr. Sebi Diet starter kit where you are furnished with step-by-step plan on how to get started on the Dr. Sebi Alkaline vegan diet. Click below to get access to your free 12-page starter kit and challenge booklet.

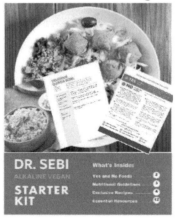

Copy the link below and paste into your browser to download
https://manage.kmail-lists.com/subscriptions/subscribe?a=X7eqXQ&g=QQnWdy

INTRODUCTION

WHY DO WE GET SICK?

We get sick because we have *deviated so much from nature*. We have let "toxins" invade and compromise our biological structure. We have let down our guards for so long. We put our bodies under chronic "stress". **Perhaps that's what the father of modern medicine, Hippocrates, meant when he said,**

> *"Illnesses do not come upon us out of the blue. They are developed from small daily sins against Nature. When enough sins have accumulated, illnesses will suddenly appear."*

So, what are these toxins? How do we get them? The toxin is our **modern food and environment.**

Many of today's diseases are **diet and lifestyle related**. And one of the reasons so many new diet fads have emerged in recent times is because we have come to realize the importance of diet and nutrition to health.

We have finally agreed that there is a problem – and we seek to fix that problem with so many diet fads. We have come to understand just how vital nutrition is for both physical and mental health. However, we have taken a misstep and gotten it wrong.

Today's science of nutrition should not only focus on calories, and nutritional facts. It should holistically look at how unnatural a diet is, gene-diet compatibility and how food intolerances contribute to certain conditions.

HOW DO WE GET SICK?

Dr. Sebi said there is no such thing as several diseases. And that the departmentalization of disease was unnecessary. There is only one disease. Whether its Leukemia, Sickle Cell anemia, or Diabetes, it's all one disease. They are not different. Apparently, what this means is that disease comes from the "same source" and is caused by an underlying factor. This factor is mucus. So, when the mucus membrane of your "biological structure is broken", then you have disease.

> *"There is only one disease – and that is a "compromising of the mucus membrane."*

Because the body is all interconnected, disease manifests in many different ways. These mucus membranes are typically violated by our acid/alkaline imbalance. When the mucus membranes are violated by acid, it results in disease.

The type of disease that manifest depends on the specific area the mucus was compromised. When the mucus at the nasal passage is compromised, it results in "sinusitis"; if at the Bronchus, it is "Bronchitis"; at the Lungs, "Pneumonia"; at the Pancreas, "Diabetes"; and at the Brain, "Alzheimer's and Parkinson's'. So, when mucus is broken down, our body systems become compromised and vulnerable to attack from disease. Dr. Sebi called it "stress". Our mucus membrane comes under undue stress which makes it penetrable to toxins that cause disease. To better under this, let us analyze the illustration below:

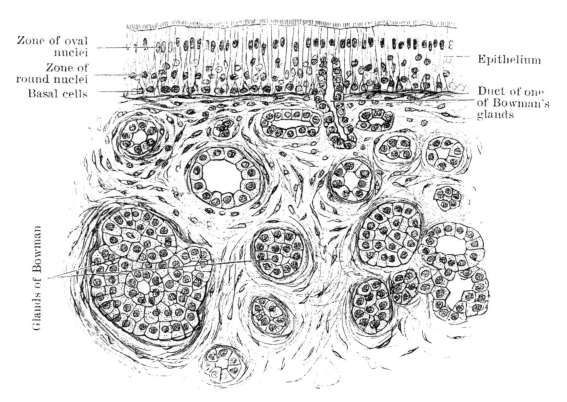

Fig: A cross-section of the mucus membrane

Visualize the mucus membrane as a guard and the acidic foods we take in as the enemy. The mucus membrane layer acts as a protective shield against the enemies of harm, germ and unwanted toxins. What happens when this layer is broken? It means our natural cellular protection has been overpowered. This is why we must do all we can to protect this membrane and the only way to do so is to maintain an alkaline state.

This theory led Dr. Sebi to conclude that total healing must focus on removing toxins and restoring energy lost by presence of disease.

THE AWAKENING

Awareness is only the first step. Execution is the second and most important step. The will and discipline to take action and follow through is sacrosanct. Understanding this basic truth is key.

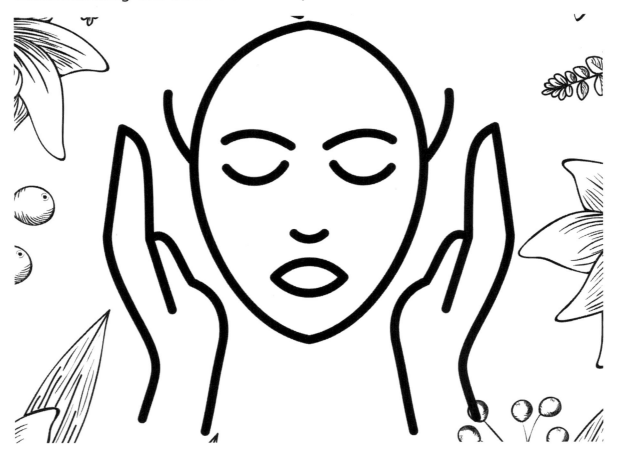

Due to an alarming increase in life-threatening diseases, most of which are diet-related and therefore preventable, more and more people have become aware of the importance of diet and are taking drastic steps to change the status quo. Even governments have intensified the promotion of natural healthy living habits both at home and at the workplace. The road to holistic healing is not in the pill, its in your food.

We now know that our body requires certain foods for optimal, holistic health. Raising awareness of the importance of a natural and healthy diet is the first step in managing your health with a diet. If your current eating habits are less than natural, being aware of what you stand to gain if you adopt a healthy diet, can serve as a powerful motivation.

A natural healthy diet is key to the following benefits:

1. *You lower the risk of many chronic diseases*
2. *You maintain a healthy blood pressure*
3. *You strengthen your immune system*
4. *You maintain healthy cholesterol levels*
5. *You have more energy*
6. *You get more focus/concentration*
7. *Your mood improves*

An electric alkaline diet is a source of energy as well as nutrients your body needs to function well. It is a natural dietary regimen that provides nutrition YOUR body truly needs to stay alive, and healthy. This diet is "live" and "electric". When your diet is electric, it will easily be absorbed by your electrical body to repair, or create new cells needed for healing. In other words, a natural electric diet enables the body to self-heal and self-repair.

It is because of this philosophy that Dr. Sebi advocated natural and holistic health. He said to avoid all unnatural foods, and blood. An important thing to be taken into consideration is that blood infers all animal or animal-based products including but not limited to meat, fish, eggs and dairy or animal seafood. And we understand this because foods such as meat and dairy are highly acidic and inflammatory, so they will create more harm than good. Also, the choice of a diet becomes particularly important if you have a chronic condition or if you are trying to prevent or heal certain diseases. Fortunately, many of the common chronic conditions can be avoided, controlled and reversed with the right diet.

CHAPTER 1:

THE DR. SEBI ALKALINE DIET

Dr. Sebi (real names: Alfredo Darrington Bowman) was a Honduran herbalist, naturalist and healer. Although, he didn't have formal medical training, he helped a lot of people cure the most serious health conditions. His secret was an alkaline electric based diet and herbal remedies. Dr. Sebi developed his healing methodology after an herbalist in Mexico helped him cure him of asthma, diabetes, and impotence. Although he had some basic knowledge of herbalism, it was after the visit to the Mexican herbalist that made him realize that even the most serious health conditions could be avoided or treated with a change of diet and herbal remedies. He has helped quite a lot of people who were written off by conventional medicine.

Dr. Sebi spent decades studying the plants and herbs of North, South and Central America, Africa and the Caribbean. Born in 1933, Dr. Sebi learned from his grandmother, "Mama Hay," and subsequently, in curing himself of diabetes, asthma, and impotency with a herbalist in Mexico. After getting healed through herbs, Dr Sebi created his unique line of natural cell food compounds that he used for cleansing and revitalization. Dr. Sebi's approach to disease relies on the theory of the African bio-mineral balance. He relies on herbal remedies to cleanse and detoxify the body, returning it to its previous intended alkaline state – a state which is free from disease.

When his healing method became well known world-wide, Dr. Sebi opened up healing practices first in Honduras, followed by New York and Los Angeles. However, because he did not have a license to practice as a healer, New York charged him with a criminal charge of working without a license. He was acquitted but was soon sued again for claiming he had a cure for AIDS, cancer, leukemia, lupus, and other untreatable diseases. In 2016 Dr. Sebi was arrested in Honduras but after falling sick while in prison and not receiving adequate treatment, he died of pneumonia-related complications. Dr. Sebi's methodology is based on an alkaline diet and healing methodology which he termed "The African Bio-Mineral Balance". His remedies are mainly based on herbs from North America, Central and South America, Africa, and the

Caribbean.

DR. SEBI ELECTRIC DIET VS CONVENTIONAL ALKALINE DIET

The concept of the alkaline diet is not a new one. It's been known since the middle of the 19-th century. Although some of the aspects of the alkaline diet were used by many nutritionists and holistic practitioners, the alkaline diet became popular relatively recently. It was during the 1990s, that some nutritionists started suggesting a 100% alkaline diet. Dr. Sebi took this a step further. He developed a diet that revolved around maintaining vitality by using the "African Bio Mineral Balance". Dr. Sebi referred to his method as either the African Bio-mineral balance or the African Bio Balance. The African Bio-mineral Balance remedy consists of 102 minerals that support electrical activity and overall vitality of the body. This therapeutic approach addresses disease on two levels. It first cleanses the body of acidity. This step relies heavily on herbs that clean the body's cells on both the cellular and intra-cellular level. The next step is to revitalize cells by supplying minerals that have been lost through the consumption of acidic foods.

Unfortunately, 90% of the modern diet is based on acidic foods, e.g. meat, dairy, processed foods as well as GMO and hybridized foods. Eating these foods will acidify the body and unbalance the alkalinity of the blood. The reason Dr. Sebi insisted on unhybridized fruits and vegetables is that such foods have an alkaline base. They were designed by nature to provide a human body with all it needs for optimal health. Dr. Sebi developed his approach to health on the assumption that disease can only exist in an acidic environment. The body works non-stop to maintain a 7.4 pH level in the blood. When you eat a balanced diet, your body is perfectly capable of maintaining this level of acidity. However, the modern diet is very unbalanced. It is based on carbs, meat, sugar, and junk food which are all very acidic and which is why our body needs help to maintain homeostasis.

Some of the cleansing herbs Dr. Sebi used in his alkaline diet are burdock root, sarsaparilla, and dandelion, which clean the blood and the liver. Dr. Sebi diet revolves around three principles that are simple to follow and that everyone can easily fit into their lifestyle, no matter how hectic or unusual.

DR. SEBI REMEDIES AND RECIPES

In this section, you will learn how to use the powerful alkaline herbs discussed earlier in this book to treat a wide variety of common ailments. Dr. Sebi believed so much in alkaline herbs that are electrical. Electric Herbs are medicinal plants which helps the human body to heal, rebuild and nourish itself. They are alkaline and found in nature. They are not hybrid, irradiated, or genetically-modified. Electric herbs improve the electrical activity in the nerves and helps with better cognitive function. It boosts your mental clarity and use of one's senses. Electricity is the reason the human body can move - crawl, walk, climb or run. Without electricity, there would be no movement and no life. If the body is electric, then you should feed it electric (alkaline) nutrition. Electric herbs are herbs made in nature, non-hybridized and non-GMO. Electric herbs are wildcrafted, grown without the use of chemical fertilizers and pesticides.

ABSCESS AND GINGIVITIS

REMEDIES

HERBAL MOUTHWASH

This powerful antimicrobial mouthwash can help fight bacteria that lead to gingivitis, as well as treat sores in the mouth. This can be created with a combination of sage and pau d' arco.

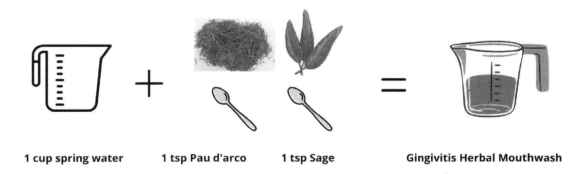

1 cup spring water   1 tsp Pau d'arco   1 tsp Sage   Gingivitis Herbal Mouthwash

Ingredients:

- 1 teaspoon Sage
- 1 teaspoon Pau d' arco
- 1 cup spring water

Directions:

1. Start by boiling two cups of water on the stove.
2. Add one teaspoon of sage and one teaspoon of pau d' arco bark. Let this simmer for ten to fifteen minutes or until the liquid is reduced by half.
3. Remove it from heat and set it aside to cool a little. When it is still warm, add one teaspoon of sea salt or Himalayan salt.
4. Blend until the salt has dissolved into the mixture. Let this cool completely and strain everything out into a glass jar for storage.
5. Store this in the refrigerator between uses.

Tip: For oral care or for treating oral sores, gargle one teaspoon of this mouthwash for two minutes. Repeat this up to three times daily until the sore has healed. For oral maintenance, gargle once daily.

SKIN ABSCESS FIGHTING TEA

Skin abscesses are often the result of a bacterial infection under several layers of the skin's surface. Oftentimes, these happen in areas of the body that are bothered by constant pressure or clothing that rubs the area a lot. Pay attention to your body and any areas that feel sore. If you feel a skin abscess in common areas like around the waist (where pants rub) or the bra line (for women it is very common to get abscesses in this area because undergarments rub it) take action right away to treat it. If an abscess is left untreated, it can develop into a much more severe infection and require lancing, which can be very painful.

You can take care of an abscess without resulting to a painful procedure with a tea made form yellow dock root. Yellow dock roots are very detoxifying and purifying. They can cleanse the body from the inside out.

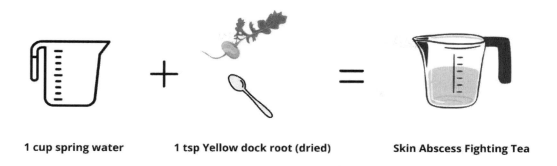

Ingredients:

- 1 teaspoon Yellow dock root, dried
- 1 cup spring water, hot

Directions:

1. Infuse one teaspoon of dried yellow dock root into one cup of hot spring water.
2. Let this infuse for up to ten minutes.
3. Drink up to three cups daily to promote the elimination of bacteria from the abscess.

Pro Tip: Use this treatment in conjunction with the next treatment for abscesses.

TOPICAL WASH FOR ABSCESSES AND GINGIVITIS

Take on an abscess of any form of bacteria with an antimicrobial and antibiotic topical wash made from yarrow and Cordoncillo negro leaves. Both of these herbs help to kill bacteria and treat skin issues that result from bacterial infections.

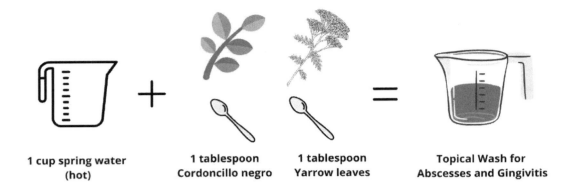

Ingredients:

- 1 tablespoon Yarrow leaves, dried
- 1 tablespoon Cordoncillo negro leaves, dried
- 1 cup spring water, hot

Directions:

1. Make a strong decoction with these to by boiling three cups of water on the stove
2. Add one tablespoon each of dried yarrow and Cordoncillo negro leaves.
3. Reduce the heat to simmer and let this infuse for up to twenty minutes.
4. Try to get the liquid to reduce by at least half.
5. Allow the liquid to cool. Strain it out when it has cooled and store it in a glass jar.
6. Refrigerate it between uses.

Prot Tip: In the refrigerator, it should last up to three weeks. You can use this in two ways. The first way is to use it for compresses on the affected area. This is very helpful for treating an abscess. Soak a small clean rag in the liquid and apply it to the area as needed until the abscess is gone. For gingivitis, simply gargle the liquid for one minute up to three times daily, depending on the severity of the case.

ACNE

REMEDIES

SKIN TONER

For a gentle yet effective skin toner that works under the surface of the skin to kill the bacteria that lead to acne, try a skin toner made with chamomile and sage. Sage kills bacteria that lead to acne and chamomile reduces redness and evens out skin tone. Together, these two herbs are the perfect combination for creating a clear complexion.

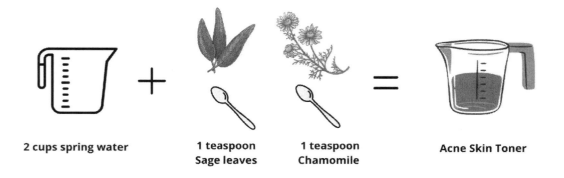

2 cups spring water + 1 teaspoon Sage leaves + 1 teaspoon Chamomile = Acne Skin Toner

Ingredients:

- 1 teaspoon Sage
- 1 teaspoon Chamomile
- 2 cups spring water

Directions:

1. Start by boiling one teaspoon each of sage and chamomile in two cups of water.
2. Reduce heat and let this simmer until the liquid is reduced to one half of a cup.
3. Strain this out and let it cool.
4. Add one fourth of a cup of raw, organic apple cider vinegar to the sage and chamomile decoction. Apple cider vinegar works well to tone and nourish the skin.
5. Stir this until the two liquids are blended.

6. Add some to a spray bottle and gently mist your clean face up to twice daily. Store this in the refrigerator between uses.

FACIAL STEAM

One of the best ways to combat acne, as well as many other skin issues, is to promote clean pores with a facial steam. Soursop leaves are perfect for an acne facial steam because they are anti-inflammatory and antimicrobial. This means they can help reduce redness and inflammation of the facial skin while also killing bacteria that cause acne.

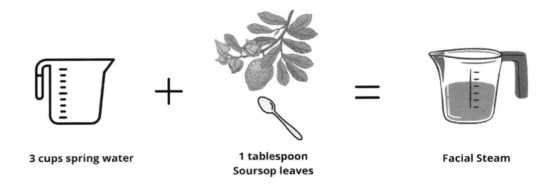

Ingredients:

- 1 tablespoon Soursop leaves, dried
- 3 cups spring water

Directions:

1. Add one tablespoon of dried soursop leaves to three cups of water on the stove and bring this to a boil.
2. Remove the pan from heat before the facial treatment to prevent being burned on the oven burner.
3. Put your face over the pan and into the steam, but take care not to get it too close, as you don't want to burn your skin.
4. Place a towel over your head to trap in steam so it can envelop your face better. Do this for fifteen minutes daily to cleanse pores and soothe the skin.

ACNE-FIGHTING TEA

Beautiful skin starts on the inside. Oftentimes, bad skin is the result of a bad diet. If you struggle with acne, avoid dairy products because they tend to affect the skin. In addition, avoid processed foods and sugars. Cleansing and purifying your body can help treat and prevent acne by flushing out the toxins that cause issues. Yellow dock root is one of the best herbs for this. It is purifying and detoxifying.

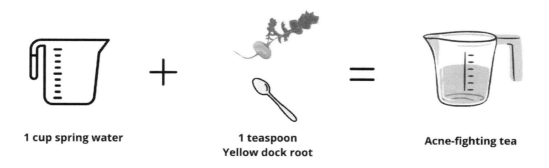

1 cup spring water   1 teaspoon Yellow dock root   Acne-fighting tea

Ingredients:

- 1 teaspoon Yellow dock root, dried and chopped
- 1 cup spring water, hot

Directions:

1. Try infusing one teaspoon of chopped and dried yellow dock roots into one cup of hot water for ten to fifteen minutes.
2. Drink this up to twice daily for detoxification and purification. Clean up your diet and try to eat more leafy greens as well. If you can do this, you will start to notice your skin glowing with health and vibrancy.

ACNE WASH

Pau d' arco is an excellent antimicrobial and antibiotic bark, making it perfect for external use treating acne.

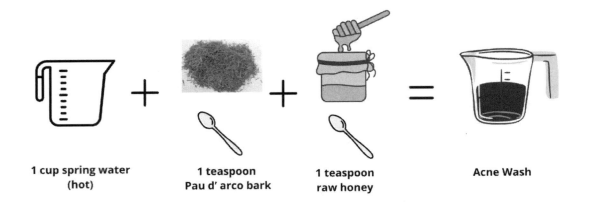

Ingredients:

- 1 teaspoon Pau d' arco bark, dried
- 1 cup spring water, hot
- 1 teaspoon raw honey

Directions:

1. Create an infusion with this bark by adding one teaspoon of the dried bark to one cup of hot water.
2. Let this infuse for fifteen to twenty minutes. Add one teaspoon of raw honey when the liquid is still warm (but not hot or it will kill the medicinal components in the honey). Allow this to blend into it well. Raw honey is highly antimicrobial and can further help to kill bacteria on the skin's surface. Soak a clean cloth into this mixture and wring it out.
3. Gently wash your clean face with this wash two to three times a day to keep your skin healthy and bacteria-free. This makes enough for several uses, just be sure to store the remainder in the refrigerator between uses.

AGING

REMEDIES

ANTI-AGING TEA 1

The key to keeping skin young is to nourish it with antioxidants. Antioxidant herbs can help to fight free radicals on the skin, which are known for causing damage and aging. A great antioxidant herb to start with is burdock root. This root is utilized in herbal medicine for its powerful antioxidant effects.

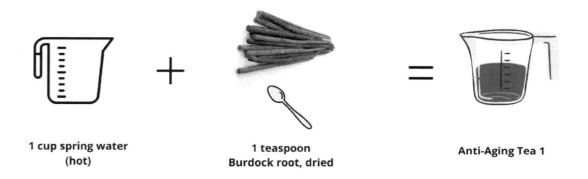

Ingredients:

- 1 teaspoon Burdock roots, dried and chopped
- 1 cup spring water, hot

Directions:

1. Infuse one teaspoon of dried and chopped burdock roots into one cup of hot water and let this sit for ten minutes before consuming.
2. Drink one cup daily to keep your skin looking youthful and radiant.

ANTI-AGING TEA 2

Irish Sea Moss is packed full of vitamins and minerals, making it a favorite among those who wish to keep young and healthy.

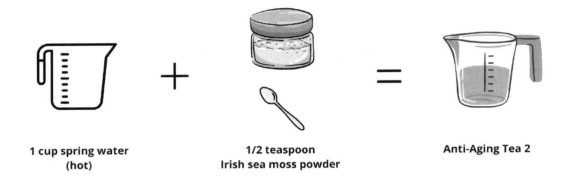

Ingredients:

- ½ teaspoon Irish sea moss powder
- 1 cup spring water, hot

Directions:

1. Infuse one half of a teaspoon of Irish Sea moss powder into one cup of hot water and let his blend together well.
2. Drink one to two cups of this today to nourish your body and integumentary system with vital nutrients that help promote healthy and vitality.
3. Irish Sea moss can also be made into a paste by adding a small amount of water to a teaspoon of the powder. Blend this until it reaches a paste-like consistency and spread it evenly on the facial skin. Leave it for fifteen to twenty minutes before rinsing off to give your skin a boost.

ALLERGIES

REMEDIES

ALLERGY RELIEF TEA

For a daily tea that helps to cleanse the blood and relieve the buildup of histamines that lead to allergies, try sarsaparilla. Sarsaparilla is excellent for allergies because it also lowers inflammation in the body. Inflammation is a major issue for those who suffer from allergies.

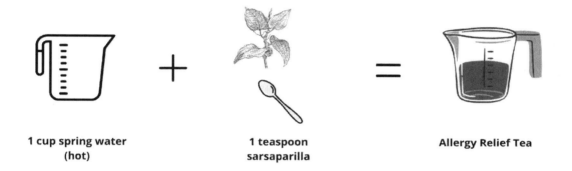

Ingredients:

- 1 teaspoon sarsaparilla
- 1 cup spring water, hot

Directions:

1. Infuse one teaspoon of sarsaparilla into one cup of hot water and let this sit for ten minutes before consuming.
2. Drink this daily to keep the blood purified and inflammation at bay.

QUICK ALLERGY TEA

Quercetin is a compound found in certain plants and herbs that works fast to target inflammation and allergies. There are many plants that contain this beneficial compound, but one of the best and most common are elderberries.

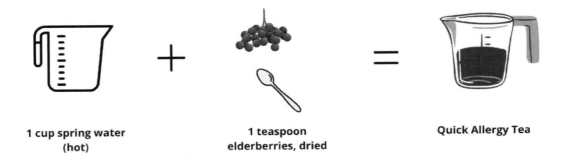

Ingredients:

- 1 teaspoon elderberries, dried
- 1 cup spring water, hot

Directions:

1. Make a strong tea with dried elderberries by infusing one teaspoon in one cup of hot water for fifteen minutes.
2. Drink up to three cups of this tea daily to help fight allergy symptoms like nasal congestion and inflammation, as well as excess mucous.

FLOWER DECOCTION

Linden flowers are excellent for calming the mind and body, but they can also lower inflammation, making them ideal for allergies. When suffering from allergies, the mucous membranes often become inflamed and can worsen symptoms. Prevent this with a decoction made from linden flowers.

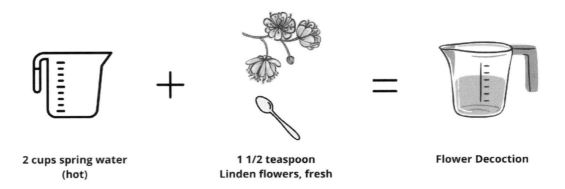

Ingredients:

- 1½ cup linden flowers, fresh
- 2 cups spring water

Directions:

1. Boil two cups of water on the stove and add one half cup of fresh linden flowers or one fourth cup of dried linden flowers.
2. Let this simmer until the liquid is reduced to one cup.
3. Remove this from heat and allow it to cool a little before consuming.
4. Drink one cup of this daily to lower inflammation from allergies.

NETTLE TEA

Stinging nettle contains flavonoids that help to lower histamine production in the body. This is great news for those with allergies, as histamines are to blame for allergy symptoms and the response the body has to allergens.

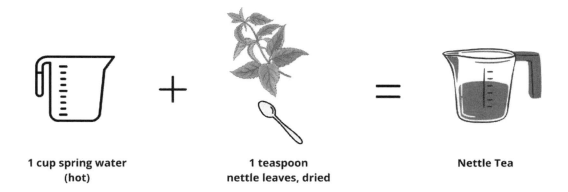

1 cup spring water (hot) + 1 teaspoon nettle leaves, dried = Nettle Tea

Ingredients:

- 1 teaspoon Stinging nettle leaves, dried
- 1 cup spring water, hot

Directions:

1. Infuse one teaspoon of dried stinging nettle leaves in one cup of hot water and let this sit for seven minutes before consuming.
2. Drink one cup daily for maintenance or three cups daily for severe allergies.

ANEMIA

REMEDIES

ANEMIA TEA

Anemia can occur when the body has low iron levels. Thankfully, there is a very common alkaline herb that naturally contains high levels of iron. This herb is the dandelion. The root of the dandelion is often used for blood cleansing and purification, but it is also a valuable source of iron for those in need of higher iron levels to treat anemia.

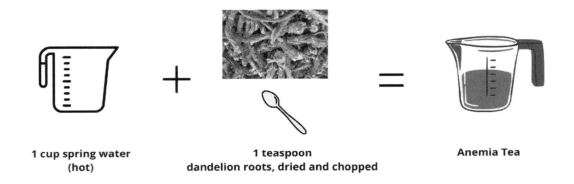

1 cup spring water (hot) + 1 teaspoon dandelion roots, dried and chopped = Anemia Tea

Ingredients:

- 1 teaspoon dandelion roots, dried and chopped
- 1 cup spring water, hot

Directions:

1. Create a tea for anemia by infusing one teaspoon of dried and chopped dandelion roots in one cup of hot water.
2. Let this infuse for at least ten minutes to ensure the iron is getting into the tea sufficiently.
3. Drink one to two cups of this tea daily to help increase iron levels and cleans the blood.

ARTHRITIS

REMEDIES

ARTHRITIS MILDING TEA

Kalawalla makes a great addition to a daily routine for the management of arthritis, especially rheumatoid arthritis. It works to balance the immune system and help keep it from attacking the body. It is great for a variety of autoimmune conditions for this reason.

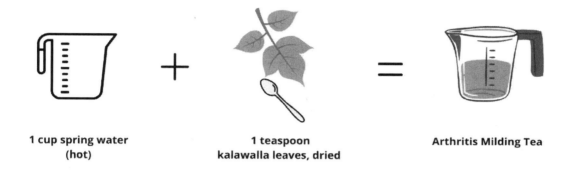

Ingredients:

- 1 teaspoon kalawalla leaves, dried
- 1 cup spring water, hot

Directions:

1. Infuse one teaspoon of dried kalawalla leaves in one cup of hot water for seven minutes before consuming.
2. Drink one cup daily to keep the immune system balanced and prevent immune system attacks on the joints.

QUICK ANALGESIC ARTHRITIS TEA

Chaparral is highly anti-inflammatory and analgesic, making it ideal for treating pain from arthritis. It you happen to find yourself in need of quick relief, try making a strong tea with chaparral.

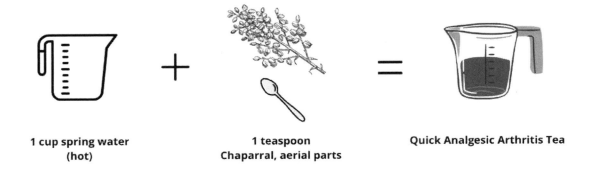

Ingredients:

- 1 teaspoon Chaparral, aerial parts
- 1 cup spring water, very hot

Directions:

1. Infuse one teaspoon of the aerial parts of the plant into one cup of very hot water. Let this sit and infuse for ten to fifteen minutes.
2. Drink this when it has cooled enough to comfortably consume.
3. Drink up to two cups of this daily for arthritis pain relief. Try using the arthritis ointment detailed below in conjunction with this remedy for maximum pain relief.

NIGHTLY ARTHRITIS TEA

Valerian root isn't just great as a sleep aid. It is a powerful analgesic and can help soothe painful joints while helping you get a good night's sleep. Valerian is a Central Nervous System (CNS) depressant. This means it slows neurotransmitter activity. One might assume this is a bad thing, but it can be a really good thing when it comes to slowing down the mind and body to prepare for sleep. In addition, this causes pain receptors to slow and results in less pain.

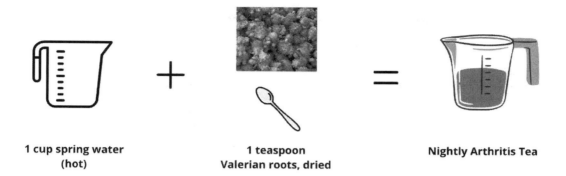

Ingredients:

- 1 teaspoon Valerian root, dried
- 1 cup spring water, hot

Directions:

1. Try infusing one teaspoon of dried valerian root in one cup of hot water for five to seven minutes before consuming.
2. Consume this tea one hour before bedtime.

ARTHRITIS OINTMENT

Soursop leaves can be used externally to bring relief to arthritic joints. They work to reduce inflammation that results from arthritis. Reducing inflammation means reducing pain in the area. These leaves can be applied like a poultice to the areas, or you can make an ointment to use any time you need it.

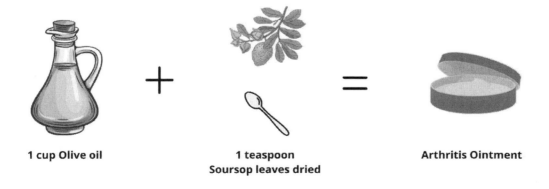

Ingredients:

- 1 teaspoon soursop leaves, dried
- 1 cup Olive oil

Directions:

1. To do this, start by infusing dried soursop leaves in a carrier oil. Olive oil makes a great carrier oil for this, as it is nourishing to the skin and can soothe any skin issues caused by arthritis. Let this infuse for four to six weeks in a dark place.
2. Shake your soursop and oil blend daily to promote further infusion.
3. After four to six weeks, strain out the oil and put eight ounces of this in a double boiler. Under low heat, add one ounce of beeswax (preferably grated beeswax or beeswax pellets). Let the beeswax melt into the oil infusion completely and then turn off the heat.

Pro Tip: You may choose at this time to add ten to twenty drops of essential oils like eucalyptus. These helps manage pain. Pour the ointment into jars to cool. When it cools, it will take on a salve-like consistency that is easy to apply to any area you choose and stays in place. Use this ointment as often as you need for relief from sore muscles, joints, and areas of trauma. As with any salve, avoid getting it in the eyes or mucous membranes.

ASTHMA

REMEDIES

QUICK ACTING ASTHMA TEA

If you find it hard to take a deep breath and are in need of quick relief, you can create a tea that can help to calm the body and open the airways fast. Two alkaline herbs that help with this are mullein and eucalyptus. Mullein is great for clearing the airways of mucous, especially the bronchial passages. Eucalyptus also helps to open the airways and promote respiratory health. It contains a constituent called 1,8 cineole that has been shown in studies to decrease anxiety before operations, which means it may help to calm the body when it is experiencing issues with asthma as well.

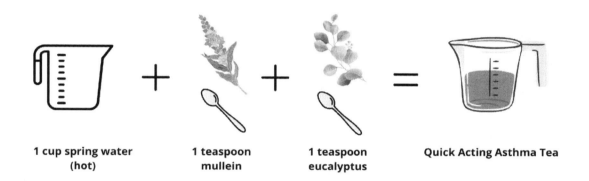

1 cup spring water (hot) + 1 teaspoon mullein + 1 teaspoon eucalyptus = Quick Acting Asthma Tea

Ingredients:

- 1 teaspoon Mullein
- 1 teaspoon eucalyptus
- 1 cup spring water, hot

Directions:

1. Combine one teaspoon each of mullein and eucalyptus in one cup of very hot water. Let these infuse for at least five minutes.
2. While you are waiting, it helps to lean down and inhale the steam coming off the tea. This can open airways and calm the body, even before you consume it.
3. When it has sufficiently cooled, consume the tea, pausing between sips to focus on breathing. Do this as often as needed to cope with asthma.

SOOTHING TEA

To soothe the body and calm spasmodic issues with the lungs and airways, try a tea made with mugwort. Mugwort is antispasmodic and anti-inflammatory, making it ideal for treating asthma or related conditions of the respiratory system. Its nervine properties mean it can calm anxiety that leads to asthmatic conditions. If you feel like you are stressed or overwhelmed, these may trigger an asthma attack. When you start to feel this way, make a cup of mugwort tea.

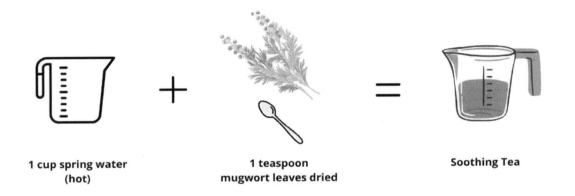

Ingredients:

- 1 teaspoon mugwort leaves, dried
- 1 cup spring water, hot

Directions:

1. Infuse one teaspoon of dried mugwort leaves into one cup of hot water for up to seven minutes.
2. Consume this when it has cooled sufficiently. You can drink up to two cups daily, as needed, for soothing relief from asthmatic conditions.

AUTISM

REMEDIES

AUTISTIC TREATMENT

Detox the body of mucus by proper blood flow that supply oxygen to the brain. It is a neurological condition. The brain works differently, and in the case of epilepsy there is abnormal nerve cell activity in the brain.

DIETARY CHANGES

Try dietary changes to control symptoms like seizures and to decrease environmental stimuli for autism. Stick to only Dr. Sebi approved foods.

A feature of Autism is the stripping away of the shell around neurons & the loss of copper (the electrical conducting metal) in the brain & nervous system. I would try to replace that metal by supplementing their diet with copper or if you can get your hands on it, monatomic gold.

Back Pain

Remedies

Spine's Fine Tincture

Mullein is often known for the medicinal properties in its leaves and flowers. However, mullein root holds a powerful medicinal secret: it can soothe spasmodic conditions relating to back and spine pain. It is an excellent remedy for any musculoskeletal issue, ranging from back muscles to a bruised coccyx. The root is best prepared in a tincture for spine pain. Start by harvesting mullein roots and chopping them. Fill a glass jar with the chopped roots and then completely cover them in at least 80 proof alcohol. Let this sit and infuse for four to six weeks. Keep this out of direct sunlight and in a cool, dark place while it infuses. Shake this daily (make sure the lid is on good) to help the mullein root further infuse into the alcohol solvent. After four to six weeks, strain out the tincture and bottle it. It is best to store tinctures in dropper bottles if possible. Take two to three droppers full as needed when you are feeling back pain coming on.

Warming Compress

Sometimes one of the best ways to combat back pain is by using a warming compress. The heat, blended with the medicinal properties in the herbal compress, helps to gently soothe and ease away pain. Guaco leaves make an excellent remedy in a compress for back pain. Start your compress by boiling one ounce of dried guaco leaves in three to four cups of water on the stove. Turn down the heat and let this simmer for fifteen to twenty minutes. Take the pot off of heat and set it aside to cool. Let this cool enough to where it doesn't hurt when the liquid is applied to the skin. When the liquid is still warm, soak a clean rag in it until it is fully soaked. Wring it out a little and place it on your back where you are experiencing pain. Let this sit on the area for as long as you can. Try lying down on your stomach when you are treating yourself with this remedy. Repeat as often as needed.

Sciatic Pain Tea

Sciatic pain comes from a nerve called the sciatic nerve. This nerve goes from your lower back through the hips to the leg. When it is aggravated, it can cause a shooting pain that radiates through these areas. To effectively tackle pain in this nerve, you will need herbs that act on the nerves. These are called "nervines." Some effective nervine herbs include blue vervain and mugwort. They act on the nervous system to calm the nerves and reduce pain. They can help with pain, inflammation, and tension as well. To make this nervine tea, combine one teaspoon each of blue vervain and mugwort and infuse them in one cup of hot water for up to seven minutes. Consume this when it is cool enough to comfortably drink. Drink one to two cups daily for help with nerve pain and spasms.

ANALGESIC DAILY TEA FOR BACK PAIN

A tea made with chamomile and elder is ideal for pain relief when it comes to back pain, spasms, and inflammation. Elderberry is very anti-inflammatory and can help reduce any inflammation that may be leading to pain. Chamomile is antispasmodic and calming. It can help reduce any tension that is causing pain. Together, these two alkaline herbs are perfect for back pain caused by inflammation and/or tension. They are gentle enough to use in a daily tea for overall health. To create this healing tea, combine one teaspoon each of chamomile flowers and dried elderberries. Let them infuse in one cup of hot water for seven to ten minutes before consuming. Drink one cup daily to support and nourish your back.

SOOTHING BACK PAIN TEA

Hops and blue vervain are known for their effect on the body and mind. Hops (also called lupulo) are sedative and anti-inflammatory. They can calm tension, as well as reduce inflammation that causes back pain. Blue vervain works on the nerves to calm spasms, reduce pain, and calm tension. Together, these provide soothing support for those experiencing any kind of back pain. Add one teaspoon of each herb to a tea bag and let this infuse in one cup of hot water for five to seven minutes before consuming. Do this daily for back pain and inflammation maintenance, or as needed when you are experiencing extra tension and stress due to back pain.

BEDSORES

REMEDIES

BEDSORE TOPICAL WASH

Bedsores result when skin becomes damaged due to decreased blood flow to the area over a period of time. This usually happens when someone is immobile and cannot move to circulate blood to all areas of the body as it should. Damaged skin from poor circulation to the area will appear as an ulcer on the skin or an infected, inflamed area. They are often sore and very painful. Alkaline herbs to treat these include chickweed and yarrow. Chickweed will provide soothing relief to the area, helping to reduce redness and inflammation. Yarrow helps to cleanse the wound and promote healing. These two works synergistically to tackle bedsores in different ways. Create an effective topical wash with chickweed and yarrow to treat bedsores by first boiling two to three cups of water on the stove. Add one ounce each of chickweed (preferably fresh) and yarrow (leaves and flowers if possible). Reduce heat and let this simmer for twenty minutes, or until the liquid is reduced by half. Wait until this has completely cooled before using it. You can use it in two ways: as a topical wash or compress. For a topical wash, simply wash the bedsores with this liquid up to five times daily. For a compress, soak a clean rag in the liquid and place it on the affected areas twice daily. In between compresses, wash and cleanse the wounds with the liquid as well. If at all possible, try to get movement and circulation to the area by moving the body as much as possible. A poultice of raw honey also works on bedsores to cleanse and heal the wounds, and is especially effective when used in conjunction with the topical wash.

Bites and Stings

Cooling Compress

For insect bites or stings that cause red, irritated skin, try a cooling compress with chickweed. Infuse one teaspoon of chickweed in one cup of hot water and make a tea, allowing this to infuse for twenty to thirty minutes and cool as it infuses. When it is completely cooled and at room temperature, soak a clean cloth in this liquid and apply it directly to the bite or sting. Let this sit as long as possible and reapply as needed.

BUT BITE RELIEF SPRAY

A bug bite relief spray is extremely handy to have when you are hiking, camping, or outdoors. It is easy to apply and very effective at reducing irritation, inflammation, and killing any germs that came into the body through the bite. To create this, boil two cups of water on the stove and add one ounce each of yarrow and yellow dock leaves. Yarrow helps kill germs and reduce infection in the area. Yellow dock cleanses the area and reduces irritation and soreness. Let this simmer for twenty minutes or until the liquid is reduced by half. Strain out the liquid and pour it in a bowl. Add one half cup of rubbing alcohol and one half cup of aloe vera juice. Blend these ingredients together well. Pour this into a spray bottle and use it as needed to treat bug bites, stings, and other wounds you may get while outdoors.

TOPICAL WASH FOR BITES AND STINGS

Contribo has been used topically for centuries to treat bites and stings, especially from poison insects or animals. It can fight any infection and kill any germs that may lead to issues. A topical wash that cleanses and detoxifies the area is optimal when you experience a bite or sting. You can create a wash with contribo leaves for this purpose. Boil two cups of water on the stove and add one tablespoon of contribo leaves. Let this simmer until the liquid is reduced by half. When this has cooled, wash the area thoroughly with this. Repeat the wash up to four times daily as needed to cleanse and heal a bite or sting.

SKIN SOOTHING OINTMENT

An ointment can be made to treat bug bites and stings that helps to reduce inflammation and redness, as well as promote healing and healthy skin. The alkaline herbs that work together in this ointment include yarrow, chickweed, and Shepard's purse. Yarrow and Shepard's purse have been used throughout history to treat wounds, and are especially helpful when it comes to cleansing and healing irritated skin from a bite or sting. Their antimicrobial properties work to cleanse and prevent infection in the area. Chickweed reduces inflammation and provides a soothing, cooling sensation. Combine one part of each herb (dried) in a glass jar and cover them with a carrier oil like olive oil. Let this sit and infuse for four to six weeks, keeping it out of direct sunlight. After four to six weeks, strain out the oil infusion and put eight ounces of this in a double boiler under low heat. Add one ounce of beeswax pellets or shavings and let this melt thoroughly. You can add essential oils like lavender or tea tree to further maximize the healing power of this ointment. If you decide to use oils, use ten to fifteen drops for an effective ointment. Pour this mixture into jars to cool and apply this ointment as needed to heal bites and sting, as well as calm the skin.

BRONCHITIS

REMEDIES

FIRE CIDER

Fire cider is an age-old remedy that employs heat from a variety of natural herbs to target viruses and infections. There are many different recipes for fire cider in different regions of the world, but many contain the following ingredients: turmeric, ginger, onion, garlic, cayenne peppers, jalapeno peppers, horseradish root, rosemary, thyme, sage, and lemon.

This colorful creation is infused in raw, organic apple cider vinegar for maximum potency. Chop one turmeric and one ginger root, one onion, one garlic bulb, one horseradish root, three to five cayenne or jalapeno peppers, one lemon, and two to three large cuttings of fresh rosemary, thyme, and sage. Fill a glass jar with these ingredients and completely cover them in apple cider vinegar to infuse.

Let this sit in a cool, dark place for at least one month before straining it out. Take a shot glass full (one ounce) as needed when you feel like you are coming down with a virus. It will heat up the body and kill infection or pathogens that are causing sickness.

THROAT SOOTHING TEA

Sage is an herb often used for its soothing and antimicrobial properties. It comes in especially handy for throat issues. If you are experiencing any drainage that irritates the throat, try a tea made with sage. Infuse one teaspoon of sage leaves (fresh or dried) into one cup of hot water. Let this infuse for five minutes. Adding one teaspoon of raw honey to this tea maximizes the throat soothing action of the tea and further helps to heal a sore throat. Drink this up to three times daily when you have a sore throat.

SWEET SOOTHING TEA

For a soothing tea that helps to open the airways and prevents infection, try a tea made with mullein leaves and pau d' arco bark. Together, these alkaline herbs help to prevent infections like pneumonia, while soothing irritation and inflammation in the respiratory system. They will also help the body expel any excess mucous causing issues. Infuse one teaspoon each of mullein leaves and pau d' arco bark into one cup of hot water. Let this sit for seven minutes before consuming. Add raw honey to sweeten this tea, as well as provide antimicrobial action. Drink one to three cups daily to help treat bronchitis while preventing any infections that may result from the excess mucous in the airways.

Burns and Sunburns

Remedies

Burn Healing Honey

Honey works wonders for all kinds of wounds, so it is no surprise it makes an excellent sunburn treatment. Maximize the treatment by infusing soothing chickweed into the honey. After harvesting chickweed, let it wilt for twenty-four hours and then place it in a glass jar. Cover the chickweed in raw, unfiltered honey. Let this infuse indefinitely. Use it as needed by applying a small amount to the affected areas and reapplying as needed for cooling comfort and healing.

Sunburn Spray

A sunburn spray is a very effective way to reach sunburn on your back because you can get the spray to reach the area. Create a soothing spray by boiling one cup of water with one teaspoon of chickweed until the liquid is reduced by half. Blend this with one half cup of aloe vera juice. Aloe vera is one of the best cures for sunburn because it is cooling, anti-inflammatory, and restorative to the skin. Store this in the refrigerator between uses. Spray on sunburned areas for instant relief.

Burn Poultice

For burns that begin to blister, a poultice may be the best route for treatment. Create a quick poultice by grinding up fresh chickweed and add a little aloe vera juice to give it a paste-like consistency. Together, chickweed and aloe vera will provide a soothing, cooling sensation while working to heal redness, inflammation, and irritation. Apply this evenly to the affected areas and leave it on as long as possible. Repeat if possible, up to three times daily.

Immunity Strengthener

For a strong immune system, try making a glycerite or tincture with elderberries. The berries are immunomodulators, meaning they can help keep the immune system running strong and healthy. They have been shown in studies to boost the immune system when it is exposed to a virus, as well as help the body fight off viruses more effectively. To make a tincture, fill a jar with dried berries and then completely cover them in at least 80 proof alcohol. If you happen to have any cinnamon sticks, add a few to this for extra immune strengthening power. Let this site and infuse in a cool, dark place for four to six weeks. After four to six weeks, strain everything out and bottle it. Take five milliliters up to four times daily at the first sign of sickness or if you have been exposed to someone you later find out was sick. To make a glycerite, fill a jar with dried or fresh elderberries and a little cinnamon if you have it. Completely cover the elderberries in non-GMO food grade vegetable glycerin. Let this infuse for four to six weeks, shaking daily to help infuse. After four to six weeks, pour the entire contents of the jar in a pot on the stove under low heat. Let this come to a boil slowly. After it has come to a boil, reduce the heat and let this sit on low heat for up to six hours. Keep an eye on your pot and stir as needed. Let this cool and strain it out through a cheesecloth, making sure to squeeze the cheesecloth hard to get the trapped liquid out. Bottle this and take five to ten milliliters at the first sign of sickness or if you believe you have been exposed to sickness.

COLD SORES

REMEDIES

COLD SORE COMPRESS

Cold sores are the result of a virus, so antiviral herbs are required to treat them. An effective herb for the job is linden flower. Linden flowers have been effectively used to treat viruses over the span of time. They are also great for soothing the affected area and reducing redness. Create a strong decoction by boiling one ounce of linden flowers in two cups of water on the stove. Reduce the heat to simmer and let the liquid reduce to one cup. When this has sufficiently cooled, soak a clean rag in the liquid and apply it to the cold sore. Leave this on for up to one hour and reapply as needed until the cold sore is gone. If possible, sleep with a compress by lying on your back to sleep.

COLD SORE BALM

A combination of yarrow, lemon balm, and St. John's wort work together to eliminate cold sores quickly. Infuse one part of each herb in coconut oil. Warm the coconut oil first by sitting the jar in a pan of warm water. When enough has melted to cover the plant material, pour it in the jar. Next, place the glass jar of herbs and coconut oil in a pan of hot water on the stove. If you have a "warm" setting on your stove, this works perfectly. If not, try sitting it in a pan of hot water on a burner under very low heat. Let this infuse for up to twelve hours before straining it out. In a double boiler, add eight ounces of herb-infused coconut oil to one ounce of beeswax. Let the beeswax melt thoroughly and then pour the balm into jars to cool. This can easily be applied to cold sores to treat them effectively and rapidly. Each herb used attacks viruses at their source and helps to quickly heal the irritated skin. Use this balm at the very first sign of a cold sore for best results. Use it as often as you can when you feel one coming.

COLD SORE TEA

A tea made with elderflower and Echinacea can work to boost the immune system to help the body fight off the herpes virus responsible for cold sores.

Elder flowers work much like elderberries to fight viruses and infections. Echinacea helps to boost the immune system and stop a virus in its tracks. Infuse one teaspoon each of elderflower and Echinacea in one cup of hot water for five to seven minutes. Consume one to three cups daily to treat a cold sore. Use this tea in conjunction with the cold sore balm for an even faster recovery.

COLD SORE MOUTHWASH

An antiviral and soothing mouthwash made from pau d' arco and soursop leaves can help to treat, as well as prevent, cold sores. Pau d' arco is antiviral in addition to antimicrobial. Soursop leaves are highly anti-inflammatory. They can work to reduce any swelling or mouth irritation caused by cold sores. Infuse one teaspoon each of soursop leaves and pau d' arco in one cup of boiling water. Let this simmer for fifteen minutes until the liquid is reduced by half. Remove this from heat and add a pinch of sea salt or Himalayan salt. Let this dissolve into the liquid. Allow the mouthwash to cool completely before using it. Gargle fifteen milliliters for up to two minutes in your mouth to help treat cold sores. Repeat this up to three times daily. Use the cold sore balm in conjunction with this remedy for rapid healing.

CONSTIPATION

REMEDIES

BOWEL-HYDRATING INFUSION

Cascara Sagrada stands in a category by itself when it comes to constipation relief. It hydrates the bowels like no other plant can by promoting excess water in the body to be absorbed by any stool in the bowels. An increase of water in the stool causes it to increase in volume and push its way out of the body easier. You can create a gentle infusion with this plant to help with constipation by first boiling two cups of water on the stove. Set aside a glass jar filled with two tablespoons of cascara sagrada. Carefully pour the boiling water over the cascara sagrada in the jar and let this sit for one to three hours. Strain out the infusion and Drink one cup when you are in need of relief. Wait at least one hour. If you do not see any results, drink the other cup (the recipe makes two cups). Make sure to drink a lot of water when you are taking this infusion, as it pulls water from the body and may result in dehydration if you do not keep drinking water to hydrate yourself.

BOWEL-MOTIVATING TINCTURE

Sometimes the bowels can be stubborn and need something to get them moving correctly. Healthy bowels start with a healthy diet, so make sure you are eating a clean diet full of alkaline foods. Avoid processed foods and sugars. You can also help things along with a tincture made from mugwort and cascara sagrada. Fill a jar with one part cascara sagrada and two parts mugwort. Cover the plant material completely with at least 80 proof alcohol. Let this sit in a cool, dark place for four to six weeks, making sure to shake daily to help it infuse better. After four to six weeks, strain out the tincture and bottle it. Take one to three droppers full when you are feeling constipated. Wait six hours before taking more. Repeat as needed for relief from constipation.

BOWEL-SOOTHING TEA

For a tea that helps to soothe irritated bowels and an upset stomach, try infusing chamomile and sage in a cup of hot water. Use one teaspoon each of chamomile and sage and let them infuse for up to ten minutes. Chamomile is famous for its calming and soothing effects on the stomach and bowels sage is carminative as well. Try adding a little raw honey to sweeten the tea and lend its gentle healing properties to the blend. Drink one to three cups daily for help with bowel and stomach discomfort.

PURIFYING DIGESTIVE TEA

For bowels in need of cleansing and purification, use dandelion and burdock root. Dandelion root is a great tonic for the body and can help flush out toxins. In addition to the root, the leaves are a powerful bitter herb. Add one half teaspoon of dried roots and one half teaspoon of dried leaves to this tea blend. Add one teaspoon of burdock root as well. Burdock root is cleansing and purifying. It helps flush out impurities and promote healthy digestion. Infuse these herbs in one cup of hot water for up to ten minutes. Drink one to two cups of this tea as needed for digestive purification.

COUGH AND COLD

REMEDIES

LUNG LUBRICATING TEA

Sometimes a cough can leave your lungs feeling irritated, inflamed, and sore. For a tea that helps to lubricate and nourish the respiratory tract, try marshmallow root and mugwort tea. Marshmallow root is known for its ability to lubricate irritated membranes in the body. It is soothing and cooling. Mugwort's nervine and anti-inflammatory properties help to further provide relief for tired lungs. Combine one teaspoon of marshmallow root and one teaspoon of mugwort in one cup of hot water. Let this sit for ten minutes before consuming. Drink one to three cups daily to help heal and repair the lungs.

ANTITUSSIVE OXYMEL

A combination of sage and wild bergamot help to quiet a bothersome cough. When infused in honey and apple cider vinegar to make an oxymel, you have a powerful healing cough treatment. An oxymel is generally an herbal preparation made with raw honey and apple cider vinegar. It is antimicrobial, healing, and antitussive. Sage is anti-spasomdic, making it perfect for calming a spasmodic cough. Wild bergamot is native to much of North America and grows wild and in abundance in many areas. The flower heads and leaves are full of powerful therapeutic properties, including antimicrobial, anti-inflammatory, and antibiotic attributes. They have a similar chemical composition to thyme, which is also a powerful cold and cough remedy. To create an oxymel with these herbs, fill a glass jar with one part wild bergamot leaves and flowers and one part sage leaves. Fill the jar, covering the plant material halfway. Cover the plant material the rest of the way with apple cider vinegar. Shake this well and store it in a cool, dry place to infuse. Shake the jar daily to help the plants infuse into the honey and apple cider vinegar better. Let this infuse for up to one month before straining it out. Take ten to fifteen milliliters as needed to calm a stubborn cough.

COUGH SYRUP

If you are in need of a quick and effective cough syrup, this recipe is perfect. This cough syrup recipe is especially helpful for those times you wake up in the night with a cough (or someone in your household is keeping you awake with a cough) and you need to whip something together to help fast. Start by filling a small cup with one teaspoon of raw honey. Add a half teaspoon of ground ginger and a fourth teaspoon of ground cinnamon. Next, add a squeeze of lemon juice and one half teaspoon of raw organic apple cider vinegar. Blend these ingredients together well. Take ten milliliters as needed to help control a cough, soothe the throat, and fight a cold.

Soothing Cough and Cold Formula

For help with a spasmodic cough that has you feeling drained and weary, try a formula with yarrow and hops. This blend is also great for fighting a cold or virus. Yarrow is often used for viruses because it induces sweating and helps to purge the body of toxins while lowering any fever. Hops is known for its soothing and nervine properties, making it effective for calming the body and helping bring much needed rest to aid in recovery. Add one part yarrow and one part hops to a glass jar and cover half of the plant material with at least 80 proof alcohol. Cover the plant material the rest of the way with raw honey and shake this well. Store this in a cool, dry place for one month and strain it out through a strainer. Take five to ten milliliters of this formula up to four times daily as needed for help with a cough or virus that has you feeling down.

Lakota Cough and Cold Formula

The Lakota Indians used wild bergamot, or *Monarda fistulosa*, as a powerful cough and cold remedy. Studies show this plant to be highly antimicrobial and antiviral. It contains high amounts of the compound thymol, making it a strong therapeutic remedy for coughs and colds. To get the most out of this plant, try making a formula that extracts both the alcohol and water soluble properties from the plant. First, fill a jar with fresh or dried wild bergamot flowers and leaves. Cover the plant material with 80 proof alcohol and let this infuse for four to six weeks in a cool, dark place. Save some wild bergamot leaves and flowers to make a strong decoction on the stove. Boil two cups of water and add one ounce of wild bergamot. Let this simmer until the liquid is reduced by half. Strain it out and let it cool. Strain out the tincture and combine even amounts of the tincture and decoction in a jar. Add a small amount of raw honey for taste. Take ten milliliters of this formula at the first sign of sickness or coughing.

LUMBEE COUGH AND COLD FORMULA

A sacred plant that grew in the North Carolina region was highly esteemed by the Lumbee Indians. This plant is goldenseal. Today, this plant is still highly revered by herbalists and natural healers. It is a source of the healing compound berberine, which is thought to combat upper respiratory infections and many other types of infections in the body. Goldenseal is endangered or threatened in some areas of the country and should be sustainably harvested to ensure its survival. If possible, it is best cultivated for use instead of wildcrafted. To make a strong formula with goldenseal, you will need the roots and aerial parts of the plant. These both contain compounds that complement one another and help the body absorb the medicinal compounds in the plant easier. Fill a glass jar with one part roots and one part leaves from the goldenseal plant.

Completely cover the plant material with at least 80 proof alcohol and let this infuse for four to six weeks in a cool, dark place. Strain out the liquid and store this in a dropper bottle. For a cough or respiratory infection, take one to three droppers full in a glass of warm water with one teaspoon of raw honey. Repeat this as needed to treat and prevent respiratory infections.

QUICK ACTING COUGH AND COLD FORMULA

For a formula that tackles cough and congestion fast, try a combination of mullein, yarrow, and elderberry. Mullein is one of the best and most effective herbs for treating respiratory issues. It can help clear the airways and expel excess mucous. Yarrow is antimicrobial and febrifuge, making it useful for colds and viruses.

Elderberry can strengthen the immune system and help the body fight off any infection or virus. Together, these three herbs work synergistically to promote a fast recovery. Add one part mullein leaves, one part yarrow leaves, and one part elderberry to a glass jar. Cover half the plant material with at least 80 proof alcohol and cover the rest of the plant material with raw honey. Shake the formula well to blend the honey and alcohol. Let this infuse in a cool, dark place for four to six weeks, shaking it daily to promote infusion. When the four to six weeks are up, strain out the liquid and bottle it. Take five to ten milliliters as needed to combat a cough or virus.

EXPECTORATING COUGH AND COLD TEA

To get rid of the excess mucous that comes with a cough or cold, try a combination of mullein and guaco. Mullein will bring the mucous out of the airways and guaco will reduce inflammation that holds mucous in the airways, as well as relieve spasms that cause coughing. Infuse one teaspoon of mullein leaves and one teaspoon of guaco leaves in one cup of hot water for seven minutes. Add raw honey to taste (it is also good for coughs). Drink one to three dups daily to promote the removal of excess mucous from the lungs and bronchial passages.

DECONGESTANT TEA

For a tea to combat congestion, an effective combination of eucalyptus and pleurisy root can help. Eucalyptus opens the airways and promotes healthy bronchial passages. Pleurisy root has been used for centuries by indigenous people to help drain excess fluid from the lungs, preventing pneumonia and any lung infection. It is invaluable to help keep the lungs healthy and able to breathe clearly. Pleurisy root is a root from a common North American plant often called by the common name "butterfly weed." Combine one teaspoon of dried and chopped pleurisy root and one teaspoon of eucalyptus leaves. Infuse these in one cup of hot water for five to seven minutes. Drink this tea up to three times daily to keep the lungs and bronchial passages clear of fluid and mucous.

ANTITUSSIVE FLOWER TEA

For a gentle floral tea blend to combat spasmodic coughing, try elderflower and chamomile. Elderflower is antiviral and anti-inflammatory. Chamomile flowers are anti-spasmodic and nervine. They can help prevent coughing and calm the body. Infuse one teaspoon of each flower in one cup of hot water for seven minutes. Add some raw honey to make a delicious, sweet floral flavor. Drink one to three cups of this tea daily if you are in need of help to calm a cough.

Quick-Acting Mullein Cough Syrup

Mullein can be consumed medicinally in many ways, but for a cough, one of the best ways is in syrup. A cough syrup with mullein can be created by first boiling two cups of water and adding one ounce of dried or fresh mullein leaves. Let this simmer until the liquid is reduced by half. You should have one cup of mullein decoction when it is through simmering. Let this cool a little until the liquid is warm but not piping hot. Add one cup of raw honey and blend everything together well. This will create a syrup consistency. The addition of raw honey is an excellent way to further add to the demulcent and antimicrobial properties of this syrup. Syrups are ideal for a cough because they are thicker and tend to coat the throat better. Take ten to twenty milliliters of this syrup as needed for a cough. If possible, try to gargle the syrup in the back of your throat before swallowing to help it coat better.

Elecampane Cough Syrup

Elecampane is a flower in the sunflower family that has been used traditionally to help with a cough. It is especially useful for loosening phlegm so it is easier to expel from the body. It has been used for respiratory conditions ranging from tuberculosis to whooping cough. The root is the part of the plant used medicinally. To make a cough syrup with this plant, harvest the roots and chop them well. In a pot on the stove, boil two cups of water with one ounce of chopped elecampane root. Let this simmer until the liquid is reduced by half, making one cup. Let this cool to the point where it is still warm but not extremely hot. Add one cup of raw honey and blend this with the elecampane decoction well. Take ten milliliters up to four times daily for help getting stubborn mucous and phlegm out of the airways.

Horehound Lozenges

Horehound is a plant in the mint family that has been used historically to treat colds and coughs. It is a natural expectorant, meaning it can help expel mucous from the body. It has a distinctive flavor, so it has been used to make candy for hundreds of years. You can make your own horehound "candy" in the form of lozenges to treat excess mucous and coughs. To start, you will need to boil two tablespoons of horehound with one cup of water on the stove. Let this simmer until you have a half of a cup of liquid. Add one cup of raw honey to the pot and stir it in well. Keep stirring the honey and horehound decoction until you notice it start to harden to a thicker consistency. While cooking, you may choose to add a teaspoon of ground ginger or cinnamon for additional therapeutic benefits. Carefully test your honey mixture from time to time by taking a small amount on a spoon and dropping it on a piece of wax paper. If it hardens, it is time to make your lozenges. Start dropping small "lozenge-sized" amounts onto the wax paper and letting them cool. When they cool, they will harden to a lozenge-like consistency. Dust your lozenges with powdered cinnamon or ginger to keep them from sticking to one another when you store them. Suck on a lozenge as needed to help control a cough and expel mucous.

CRAMPS

REMEDIES

MUSCLE WARMING OINTMENT

For an ointment that gently warms, try creating this ointment made with cayenne and cordoncillo negro leaves. Cayenne peppers are a powerfully medicinal plant because they contain compounds that reduce inflammation and pain. The active medicinal compound in these peppers is what gives them their heat. The gently warming heat from an ointment made with cayenne provides more than just pain relief. It also helps with blood circulation in the affected area. Adding cordoncillo negro leaves to this makes an even more powerful anti-inflammatory ointment with the ability to bring relief to muscles, bring down swelling, and reduce soreness. To start, infuse one tablespoon of ground or powdered cayenne peppers into one half cup of olive oil. Do this in a double boiler. Next, add one tablespoon of chopped cordoncillo negro leaves to the oil and let this infuse under low heat for two hours. Use a spoon with holes to lift out the used cordoncillo negro leaves when the infusion is over. Finally, add one and a half tablespoons of beeswax pellets and let this melt into the oil. Remove the ointment from heat and pour it into jars to cool. Apply a liberal amount to sore muscles as needed. Avoid contact with mucous membranes and eyes when using this ointment. Wash your hands well after applying it.

MUSCLE CRAMP TEA

Eucalyptus is an alkaline herb that is known for its ability to help with muscle cramps when taken internally, as well as externally. Eucalyptus tea can help soothe sore muscles because it contains pain-relieving compounds that can treat a variety of complaints. To create a tea with eucalyptus for muscle cramps, try infusing one teaspoon of dried eucalyptus leaves into one cup of hot water for five to seven minutes. Drink two to three cups of this tea as needed to attack sore muscles from the inside out.

MUSCLE RUB

For external pain relief, eucalyptus can be made into a powerful muscle rub that treats sore muscles and joints. Start by filling a sterile glass jar with dried eucalyptus leaves. Completely cover the leaves in a carrier oil like olive oil. Sit this somewhere to infuse for four to six weeks. Shake it daily. Keep the jar out of direct sunlight to prevent damaging the plant material and making it less potent. After four to six weeks, strain out the oil and add eight ounces to a double boiler. Next, add one ounce of beeswax and let this melt under low heat. Remove the muscle rub mixture from heat when the beeswax melts. At this time, you may choose to increase the potency even more by adding ten to twenty drops of eucalyptus, peppermint, tea tree, or rosemary essential oil, but this is optional. Pour the muscle rub into jars to cool. Apply a liberal amount of this to sore muscles and joints as needed.

Diarrhea

Remedies

Astringent Tea

Yarrow is an alkaline herb that has astringent properties, making it useful to bring relief to the bowels by encouraging the healing of the intestines and tissues that are irritated. Astringent herbs tighten tissues and tone weak body tissue. When one has diarrhea, the intestines may be weak and in need of toning astringents. Additionally, astringent herbs help reduce irritation, redness, and swelling. They are often used to treat complaints like diarrhea, hemorrhoids, and inflammatory conditions. Make a gentle and soothing tea with yarrow leaves or flowers by infusing one teaspoon of yarrow in one cup of hot water for five to seven minutes. Drink two to three cups as needed for astringent healing. This tea can also be used as a wash to treat hemorrhoids. If using it as a hemorrhoid wash, cleanse the affected area up to five times daily with this tea recipe.

Cinnamon Powder Capsules

Cinnamon is a rich source of a compound called coumarin. This medicinal compound has many uses, including lowering inflammation, nourishing the heart, easing digestive woes, killing bacteria and viruses, increasing circulation, and eliminating fungal infections. For digestive complaints like diarrhea, cinnamon can help stimulate salivation and gastric juices which in turn can ease digestion. Many people opt to take cinnamon daily as a dietary supplement for many ailments, so they grind it into powder to put in capsules. It is important to note that not all cinnamon is created equal. There are two varieties: cassia cinnamon and Ceylon cinnamon. Cassia is what most people use and is more readily available at grocery stores. Ceylon is considered "true" cinnamon. It has a sweeter flavor and less coumarin. You might think that less coumarin is bad since coumarin is also what gives cinnamon its medicinal properties. However, too much coumarin is not safe because it can result in liver damage if taken over time. In higher doses, coumarin can also thin the blood too much. Ceylon has just the right amount of coumarin to be safe and effective. Place 150 milligrams of Ceylon cinnamon powder into capsules and take two daily for help with diarrhea and stomach complaints.

Quick and Easy Diarrhea Tea

An alkaline herb that has been shown to be very effective for treating diarrhea is stinging nettle. Stinging nettle not only helps replenish vital nutrients the body may be lacking from diarrhea, but it can help eliminate diarrhea and return your intestinal tract to normal. For many people with chronic diarrhea, they may find they are lacking in nutrients that keep them healthy and balanced. Stinging nettle is a rich and robust source of vitamins A, C, K, and B. They also contain valuable minerals and fatty acids. A tea made with stinging nettle is the perfect remedy to balance the body, replenish lost nutrients, and encourage a healthy intestinal tract after suffering from diarrhea. Make a strong tea so you get all the nutrients by infusing two teaspoons of stinging nettle into one cup of hot water for ten minutes. Drink these two to three times daily for the treatment and prevention of diarrhea. Make sure to drink plenty of water if you have diarrhea, as it can dehydrate the body fast.

Soothing Diarrhea Tea

Chamomile and Sage are soothing to the stomach and intestinal tract, so they are the perfect alkaline remedy for treating diarrhea, an upset stomach, gas, bloating, and a wide variety of stomach and intestinal ailments. Chamomile's soothing and anti-spasmodic properties make it perfect for calming a spasmodic gut when you have diarrhea. Sage works to calm the digestive tract as well, and can help bring quick relief when you need it. Combine one teaspoon each of chamomile flowers and sage leaves in one cup of hot water. Let this infuse for five to seven minutes before enjoying. Drink one to three cups as needed for the treatment of diarrhea, upset stomach, gas, bloating, or other similar digestive complaints.

Iroquois Tea

Agrimony is a native plant to much of North America. This beneficial plant was used by the Iroquois to treat stomach complaints and especially diarrhea. All parts of the agrimony plant were used to heal the body. This plant is easy to find in the summer months and is identified by its yellow flowers that emerge on spikes. When harvesting agrimony, try to take mostly aerial parts to give plants a chance to live. In areas where there are many, you can dig up a few roots to use medicinally as well. Process the plants by cleaning them and then laying or hanging them to dry. Store the dried plants in an airtight jar and keep them out of direct sunlight. This way you will have plenty of good quality agrimony to use when you need it. To make a tea with agrimony, grind up one teaspoon of root and aerial parts of the plant. Infuse this in a cup of hot water for seven to ten minutes before consuming it. Drink one to three cups of this tea daily or as needed for the treatment of diarrhea and other digestive complaints.

FATIGUE

REMEDIES

SHAKE-IT-OFF FORMULA

If you are being held back by mild to moderate depression, try a formula made with damiana and blue vervain to start your day. Those suffering from mild to moderate depression often report that they feel fatigued and tired a lot. They may also experience little to no motivation. Damiana can help to balance hormones that cause fatigue and depression. Blue vervain acts as a nervine to promote feelings of positivity and uplifting. Combine one part damiana and one part blue vervain in a sterile glass jar and completely cover the plant material with at least 80 proof alcohol. Let this infuse for four to six weeks in a cool, dark place. After four to six weeks, strain out the liquid and bottle it in a dropper bottle. Take two to three droppers full in the morning with food. Take one to three droppers full in the afternoon as needed to control depression, fatigue, and low motivation.

UP AND ABOUT MORSELS

Do you find it hard to get going in the morning? Many people have a hard time getting out of bed and getting their day started. You can help super-charge your body and get off to a great start with Up and About Morsels. These contain Nopal and Irish Sea Moss. Both of these are superfoods. Superfoods are foods that are packed with important vitamins, minerals, and other nutrients to give you optimal nutrition. This nutrition can help you start your day with energy and stamina in order to tackle anything that comes your way. To make these, infuse one tablespoon each of powdered nopal and powdered Irish Sea moss into one cup of organic coconut oil under low heat for one hour. Remove from heat and add one tablespoon of organic, gluten free rolled oats and one tablespoon of organic almond butter. Stir this together well. Place the bowl in the refrigerator for fifteen minutes or until you notice the coconut oil start to go back to a solid state. Before the coconut oil becomes too hard to work with, take it out of the refrigerator and stir the contents of the bowl one more time. Now take a spoonful of the mixture at a time and roll it into a small ball. Place the balls on a flat surface and sit it in the refrigerator overnight to harden completely. Enjoy a cup of these each morning to give you a protein and nutrition boost to enliven your day.

PICK-ME-UP TEA

If you find yourself needing a pick-me-up as you go about your day, try a purifying and cleansing tea made with burdock root. Burdock root can help flush out the toxins that weigh you down and make you sluggish throughout the day. Infuse one teaspoon of burdock root in one cup of hot water for five to seven minutes. Add a little raw honey to taste (and for an additional pick-me-up). Enjoy one cup of this tea in the afternoon when you feel yourself start to get tired and fatigued after a long day.

INVIGORATING TEA

Eucalyptus is a lively and invigorating alkaline herb. Its fresh and camphorous compounds help bring energy and vigor to a tired body and mind. It is often enjoyed in the aromatherapy world for its ability to bring energy and vitality just from the scent alone. Drinking it in tea can help give you the momentum you need to get your day going or the vigor to finish the day strong. In addition, it can help open up the sinuses and allow you to breathe easier and deeper. Infuse one teaspoon of eucalyptus leaves into one cup of hot water for five to seven minutes. Add a small amount of raw honey for an extra boost. Drink this in the morning or afternoon for a stimulating and revitalizing experience.

FEVER

REMEDIES

FEVER-REDUCING TEA

Yarrow is one of the most popular herbs for reducing a fever. It is known to work by inducing sweating, which helps to naturally cool the body down. You can create a gentle and effective tea for treating high fevers by infusing one teaspoon of dried or fresh yarrow leaves into one cup of hot water for five to seven minutes. Drink one to four cups daily as needed for help reducing a fever. A fever should be left alone unless it gets very high. It is the body's way of heating up to make itself inhospitable for a virus or infection. If you bring a fever down when it is not that high you are robbing yourself of this tactic that is helping to kill a virus or pathogen and heal you. A good rule of thumb is to keep an eye on a fever and take your temperature often when you feel you have a fever. Let the fever get up to 103 or 104 degrees Fahrenheit before you take action. An exception to this rule is if the fever is making you miserable and you are unable to keep food or water down because of it. Drink plenty of fluids when you have a fever to avoid dehydration, as a fever can make one dehydrated faster than normal.

FEVER-BREAKING TEA

Sarsaparilla is another alkaline herb that works to reduce a fever. It is also a great source of iron, helping to keep you strong and healthy. Create a tea with sarsaparilla by infusing one teaspoon of dried sarsaparilla into one cup of hot water for seven to ten minutes. Drink one to two cups as needed for help controlling a high fever. In addition, consider taking a tepid bath to bring a fever down. Another helpful action you can take to help with a fever is to place a cool compress on the forehead or neck area.

Fever Relief Tea

Contribo is known for helping the body fight off viruses or other pathogens that cause sickness. It can provide more energy when you are feeling sick, as well as increase your appetite so you can get the nutrients you need when you are feeling ill. Contribo also improves circulation and calms the digestive system, helping you to recover faster. Try consuming contribo in tea when you have a fever or illness by infusing one teaspoon of dried contribo into one cup of hot water for seven to ten minutes. Drink one to two cups daily to kick the immune system into high gear and fight off a virus or infection.

QUICK-ACTING FEVER TEA

A powerful and synergistic combination of elderberry and yarrow can help manage a fever quickly. These two herbs work to fight illness in two ways: the elderberry stimulates the immune system and helps if fight the cause of the illness while the yarrow helps lower a fever and flush out any toxins that may be causing issues. Infuse one teaspoon of yarrow and one teaspoon of dried elderberries in one cup of hot water for ten minutes. Add raw honey to taste. Drink one to four cups of this tea daily to knock out a fever fast.

FOOD INTOLERANCES

REMEDIES

GUT-HEAL TEA

Sometimes the gut becomes imbalanced and the bad bacteria take over. Keeping our microbiome healthy is of the utmost importance because much of our immune systems rely on a healthy gut biome to function properly. Slippery Elm and Cinnamon can help replenish the good bacteria while promoting regular bowel movements to keep you healthy. Infuse one teaspoon of slippery elm bark and one teaspoon of finely chopped cinnamon bark into one cup of hot water for ten minutes. Stir this well and drink one to two cups of this tea daily to manage gut health, a healthy microbiome, and digestive wellness.

BUILD-UP BROTH

Stinging Nettle is one of the best alkaline herbs for replenishing the body and providing essential nutrients. If you need built up after an illness, surgery, or diarrhea, try a nourishing broth made with stinging nettle leaves. A combination of the broth and the nutrient-dense nettle leaves will help restore the body and nurture the gut. Making your own bone broth is so much easier than most people realize. The next time you cook a turkey, chicken, beef, or any other meat with bones, try making a broth with the leftover bones. You can do this by filling a large stock pot with the bones and water. Add hearty and nutritious ingredients to the pot like garlic cloves, onions, rosemary, thyme, or sage. Add one to two cups of fresh or dried stinging nettle leaves to the pot as well. Bring the pot of water, bones, and herbs to a boil and reduce the heat to simmer. Let this simmer for as long as possible to make sure you get all the nourishing collagen from the bones and connective tissues. You can leave the pot simmering under very low heat for up to twelve hours if you want. Just make sure to keep an eye on it so it doesn't evaporate down too much. Pour the finished broth through a strainer and into jars to store. If you won't be using it right away, you can portion it out into containers and freeze some. When you need built-up, simply take some broth out of the freezer and gently re-heat it on the stove. Enjoy this as needed when you are recovering.

STOP FLATULENCE TEA

Stop uncomfortable gas and bloating with a tea made from chamomile. This alkaline herb both soothes and calms digestive discomfort that leads to gas. Chamomile also calms spasms that cause discomfort in the digestive tract. Make a calming tea by infusing one teaspoon of dried or fresh chamomile flowers into one cup of hot water for five to seven minutes. Drink one to three cups as needed to help with flatulence and digestive woes.

COLON-SOOTHING TEA

Mugwort has been used for digestive issues for centuries because it is so versatile when it comes to what this herb does for the digestive tract. It is a bitter digestive, meaning it can help manage colic, gas, cramps, constipation, diarrhea, and sluggish digestion. Mugwort makes the perfect herb for colon soothing because of all it can do. Make a comforting tea with mugwort by infusing one teaspoon of dried or fresh mugwort into one cup of hot water for five to seven minutes. Drink this daily for colon health and comfort.

QUICK-ACTING FLATULENCE TEA

Sage can help tackle irritating flatulence quick. It is known for its ability to ease bloating, gas, stomach pain, cramps, diarrhea, and even heartburn. It can help neutralize an acidic stomach fast and eliminate gas and bloating as a result. Make a strong tea with sage for fast relief. Infuse two teaspoons of dried or fresh sage into one cup of hot water for seven to ten minutes. Drink this as needed to manage an upset stomach.

GUT-CLEARING TEA

Cascara sagrada helps to encourage a bowel movement, so it is the perfect remedy for eliminating waste from the gut. Constipation is not good for the body in many ways. The waste in our gut needs to be cleared out often to maintain a healthy microbiome. If you are concerned about sluggish digestion and too much waste in the digestive tract, try a tea made with cascara sagrada. Infuse one teaspoon of cascara sagrada into one cup of hot water for ten minutes. Drink half of this and set the rest aside. Wait one hour and if you still need to have a bowel movement, drink the rest of the cup. Repeat this until you have a bowel movement. Over time, you will learn just how much of this tea you need to help clear your gut. Everyone is different when it comes to the amount that it takes to work for their needs.

DAILY DIGESTIVE TEA

Yellow Dock is a friend when it comes to aiding with digestion. It can help the body absorb nutrients better and relieve any inflammation in the digestive tract. In addition, it can work as a gentle laxative for those needing a little help eliminating waste. When consumed in a daily tea, yellow dock can encourage healthy digestion. Infuse one teaspoon of chopped (fresh or dried) yellow dock root into one cup of water for ten minutes. Consume one cup of this tea daily for best results.

PEPPERY INDIGESTION TEA

Black pepper is more than just a spicy food flavoring. It can help to aid the body in the production of digestive enzymes and juices, as well as reduce inflammation in the digestive tract. It also supports healthy circulation in the body and helps to settle an upset stomach. Ginger is also known for its ability to calm an upset stomach and reduce digestive discomfort. Together, black pepper and ginger complement each other well in a tea for indigestion. They are both pleasantly spicy, but not overpowering. Infuse one teaspoon each of chopped ginger (fresh or dried) and organic black peppercorns in one cup of hot water for ten minutes. Enjoy this tea when you need quick relief from indigestion, an upset stomach, or digestive discomfort.

HANGOVER

REMEDIES

TAKE-IT-EASY NEXT DAY INFUSION

Replenish lost nutrients from over-indulgence with a strong and nourishing infusion made with stinging nettle. A hangover can leave you dehydrated and in need of sustenance. Stinging nettles can help replace any depleted nutrients while encouraging the flushing of toxins from too much alcohol. This infusion is especially handy if you have a hangover that is causing vomiting or diarrhea. Make an infusion by boiling two cups of water on the stove. Fill a sterile glass jar with one cup of dried or fresh stinging nettle leaves. Carefully pour the boiling water into the glass jar over the stinging nettle. Allow this to sit and infuse for two hours before consuming it. Try to drink the entire infusion by drinking one cup at a time at intervals throughout the day. Drink plenty of water as well.

NO-FUSS HANGOVER TEA

Dandelion root is an effective remedy for treating a hangover because it helps flush out toxins, cleanses impurities from the body, and acts as a general tonic when you are feeling unwell. In addition, dandelion root can calm an upset stomach, something many people suffering from a hangover experience. Dandelion is very common and easy to come by, so it is an easy remedy when you are feeling down from a hangover. Infuse one teaspoon of chopped (fresh or dried) dandelion root into one cup of water for ten minutes. Add raw honey to taste. Drink one to three cups of this tea as needed to flush out your system and recover faster. Drink as much water as you can while recovering from a hangover to prevent dehydration and promote cleansing in the body.

QUICK-ACTING HANGOVER TEA

Sometimes the best cure for a hangover is to stay hydrated and get some rest. Valerian root can help you achieve a deep slumber so you can wake up feeling refreshed and ready to go. Valerian root acts quickly in the body to slow down the Central Nervous System so you can relax and get the rest your body needs. It is also analgesic, so it can calm a headache caused by a hangover. Before consuming, make sure you have consumed plenty of water. When you are ready to lie down and sleep off a hangover, infuse one to two teaspoons of (dried or fresh) chopped valerian root into one cup of hot water. Add raw honey to help with the taste. Drink this and find a comfortable spot to take a nap. When you wake up, drink more water and take it easy until you feel like yourself again.

SPICY HANGOVER TEA

Cayenne and lemon tea can recharge the body while you are recovering from a hangover. One of the best things about cayenne is that it is a natural pain reliever, so if you are suffering from a headache, it can help bring relief. Cayenne also calms an upset stomach caused by overindulgence in alcohol. The addition of lemon helps to create a more alkaline state in the body that may be offset by drinking alcohol. It can also help relieve any headache or body pains you may be experiencing as you recover. Many people assume that drinking something spicy would upset the stomach when it is already upset from a hangover. However, the truth is that cayenne can calm an upset stomach and bring relief. Gently stir one half teaspoon of ground cayenne into three fourths cup of hot water. When it is fully dissolved, add one fourth of a cup of lemon juice. Finally, add a teaspoon of raw honey. This will create a surprisingly pleasant drink to help ease any bodily distress.

HEADACHE

REMEDIES

COOLING HEADACHE TEA

For a cooling and refreshing tea that works to melt tension and reduce inflammation, combine soothing linden flower with yarrow. Linden flowers help to ease tension in the body and mind, which often contributes to headaches. Yarrow has the unique ability to lower inflammation in the head that causes restrictions on blood vessels. When these blood vessels are restricted, a headache can result. Together, yarrow and linden flowers work to get rid of a headache on different levels. Try infusing one teaspoon each of linden flowers and yarrow (leaves and flowers) in one cup of hot water for seven to ten minutes. Allow this to completely cool and drink it on ice for invigorating relief. Drink one to three cups of this tea as needed for tension headaches or headaches caused by inflammation.

WARMING HEADACHE TEA

Cayenne and ginger pair perfectly in a warming tea that can ease pain and knock out a headache. Cayenne is famous for its analgesic qualities and ginger is equally known for its ability to reduce pain and inflammation. Oftentimes, inflammation is to blame for a headache because it restricts blood flow in the head. Cayenne can help to restore circulation while ginger works to reduce inflammation, helping blood flow return to normal. Cayenne is a source of a compound called capsaicin, which is useful for activating nerve cells to reduce pain. Infuse one teaspoon of finely chopped or grated ginger (dried or fresh) with one half of a teaspoon of ground cayenne in one cup of hot water. Allow these to infuse for five to seven minutes. Stir the tea well to help the cayenne powder dissolve into the water. Consume one cup of this tea as needed to reduce pain from a headache.

PEPPERY HEADACHE TEA

Black pepper is another spicy herb that can help with pain from a headache. This is because it contains compounds that are both anti-inflammatory and analgesic. In addition, a tea made with black pepper can help calm an upset stomach caused by a migraine or headache. To make this tea, infuse one teaspoon of organic black peppercorns into one cup of hot water for five to seven minutes. For an extra anti-inflammatory and analgesic kick, try adding one teaspoon of chopped (fresh or dried) turmeric root. Both black pepper and turmeric complement one another. Black pepper can also help the body better absorb the medicinal compounds in turmeric. Drink one to two cups of this tea as needed for respite from a headache or migraine.

Soothing Headache Tea

Valerian and chamomile aren't just great for helping you relax. They also have analgesic, anti-inflammatory, and anti-spasmodic properties. This tea blend is perfect for headaches caused by anxiety, stress or other nerve issues. It can help to relax the body, relieve tension, and ease any pain in the body. It will also help you sleep off a particularly bad headache or migraine. This is best taken at the first sign of a headache or migraine. When you feel one coming on, infuse a teaspoon of chopped valerian root and a teaspoon of chamomile flowers in one cup of hot water for seven to ten minutes. Consume this and find a peaceful, dark location to take a nap or just close your eyes and meditate for a while.

Heartburn/Reflux/GERD

Remedies

Marshmallow Infusion

Marshmallow root may be just what you need to help soothe an irritated throat or esophagus. It can also help negate the acidity of the contents of the stomach, bringing much needed relief to those with heartburn or acid reflux. To make an effective infusion, start by bringing two cups of water to boil on the stove. Meantime, fill a glass jar with two tablespoons of dried marshmallow root. Carefully pour the boiling water over the marshmallow root and let this infuse for two to four hours. You want to see the liquid become somewhat thicker and attain a "smooth" consistency. After two to four hours, consume this in half-cup increments throughout the day to support an alkaline stomach and prevent or treat heartburn and reflux.

Preventative Bitter Tincture

Bitter herbs are herbs that aid in digestion and help to calm a wide variety of stomach and digestive issues. They are also perfect for daily use to prevent heartburn, acid reflux, and gastroesophageal reflux disease (GERD). Some bitter alkaline herbs include dandelion root/leaf and burdock root. These herbs are also rich sources of vitamins and minerals the body needs to stay healthy. Mugwort is another digestive bitter and can ease indigestion, bloating, gas, and more. Combine these in a tincture for a powerful way to prevent and treat a wide range of digestive discomforts. Fill a sterile glass jar with one part dandelion leaf and root, one part mugwort, and one part burdock root. Next, completely cover the plant material with at least 80 proof alcohol. Let this sit and infuse for four to six weeks, shaking the bottle daily to help it infuse better. After four to six weeks, strain out the tincture and bottle the liquid in a dropper bottle. Take two droppers full daily, spacing doses out by taking one in the morning and one in the evening. Take each dose with a little food and make sure you drink plenty of water to keep healthy and encourage proper digestion.

Quick-Acting Heartburn Tea

For quick relief from heartburn, try making a strong tea with sage. Sage can help negate acid and calm an upset stomach. It is also carminative and aids in digestion. Infuse two teaspoons of fresh or dried sage leaves into one cup of hot water for seven to ten minutes. Drink one to two cups as needed for quick relief from heartburn. Make sure to avoid foods and drinks that can trigger heartburn like tomatoes, orange juice, alcohol, onions, garlic, or spicy foods.

SOOTHING HEARTBURN TEA

Chamomile and catnip work together to soothe an irritated esophagus while reducing inflammation and settling an upset stomach. They are also perfect for calming stress or anxiety that can trigger heartburn. Combine one teaspoon each of chamomile and catnip and infuse them in one cup of hot water for five to seven minutes. Drink this tea as needed when you need relief from stress or anxiety-induced heartburn.

INDIGESTION/DYSPEPSIA

REMEDIES

PRE-EMPTIVE BITTER TINCTURE

Mugwort and dandelion are great together in a bitter tincture for preventing indigestion if you are prone to indigestion after meals. If you take this tincture before and after eating, it can help prevent issues before they have a chance to emerge. Combine one part dandelion leaf, one part dandelion root, and one part mugwort in a glass jar. Next, completely cover the plant material with at least 80 proof alcohol. Allow this to sit and infuse for four to six weeks, making sure you store it in a cool, dark place. Shake the bottle daily to get the plant material to infuse in the alcohol quicker. After four to six weeks, strain out the liquid and bottle it. Take one to two droppers full before and after each meal. Drink plenty of water and avoid overeating. Avoid foods that trigger indigestion like spicy or fried foods.

CARMINATIVE TINCTURE

Chamomile and sage pair well in a tincture to settle an upset stomach and promote digestive health. Chamomile soothes and settles the stomach while sage treats and prevents discomforts like gas, bloating, and indigestion. Combine one part sage leaves and one part chamomile flowers in a glass jar and completely cover them with at least 80 proof alcohol. Let this infuse for four to six weeks before straining out. Store the tincture in a dropper bottle and take one to three droppers full as needed to settle the stomach and calm any indigestion, gas, bloating, or digestive discomfort.

DIGESTIVE TEA

Chickweed and stinging nettle work seamlessly in this tea blend to promote healthy digestion and flush out toxins that lead to problems like infections and diarrhea. Chickweed is often used to soothe and treat skin issues because it is highly anti-inflammatory and cooling. However, it is also a nutritious edible herb that can heal the body when taken internally. Stinging nettle is a diuretic and can help the body get rid of excess water, sending it out through the bowels or urine. This flushes out unwanted toxins in the digestive and urinary tract. Combine one teaspoon each of fresh chickweed and fresh or dried stinging nettle leaves. Infuse these in one cup of hot water for five to seven minutes before consuming. Drink one cup daily for digestive maintenance.

STRONG DIGESTIVE TEA

Ginger, fennel, and catnip make a strong combination for those wishing for a strong remedy to get rid of digestive woes like gas, bloating, upset stomach, and indigestion. These herbs help promote healthy digestion and support the gentle elimination of the bowels. Ginger is anti-inflammatory, making it ideal for calming any digestive issues that lead to inflammation. Fennel is highly carminative and aids in digestion. Catnip is soothing and nourishing to the digestive tract. Combine one teaspoon each of grated ginger, fennel seeds, and catnip leaves. Infuse these in a cup of hot water for ten to fifteen minutes to create a stronger tea for treating digestive ailments. Drink one to two cups daily as needed for digestive health.

QUICK-ACTING DIGESTIVE TEA

Prodigiosa acts fast to calm issues of the digestive system such as diarrhea, stomach pain, and indigestion. Lupulo complements prodigiosa well because it works to calm the body and mind, easing tension and anxiety that leads to digestive issues. Lupulo is carminative, sedative, and anti-inflammatory. Create a tea to rapidly banish digestive woes by combining one teaspoon of dried prodigiosa and one teaspoon of dried lupulo and infusing these in one cup of hot water for ten minutes. Drink one cup as needed for timely relief.

Insomnia

Remedies

End-Of-The-Day Elixir

At the end of a long day, it can be difficult to shut off a racing mind and get ready for sleep. A gentle elixir that helps get the brain ready for sleep can help you get the rest you need. This elixir is made with blue vervain and skullcap. Blue vervain acts on the nerves to settle the body and help rein in the mind. Skullcap is a powerful nervine that can ease the nerves and calm frustration, anxiety, stress, and a feeling of being overwhelmed. This elixir will help you reset to take on the next day. Combine one part blue vervain and one part skullcap in a glass jar. Cover half of the plant material with brandy and half with at least 80 proof alcohol. Sit the jar somewhere to infuse for four to six weeks. After four to six weeks are up, strain out the liquid. Add a teaspoon or two of raw honey for taste if desired and shake well. Take one to three droppers full at the end of the day as you are preparing to go to bed. At least one hour before bed time, avoid all screens from phones, tablets, or televisions. Blue light from these screens can mess with the brain and keep the body awake longer.

Sleep Formula

Lupulo, valerian, and lemon balm combine in this powerful sleep formula to help you get to sleep fast and stay asleep. If you have trouble getting to sleep or wake up in the night restless and unable to get back to sleep, this formula is for you. Lupulo is a mild sedative and can help relax the body and mind. Valerian is one of the most effective sleep remedies for its effect on the Central Nervous System. Lemon balm is a nervine herb that can bring peace and quiet to an overwhelmed mind. Combine one part each of dried and chopped valerian roots, lupulo, and lemon balm in a glass jar. Completely cover the contents of the jar with at least 80 proof alcohol. Let this sit in a cool, dark place for four to six weeks, shaking it daily to help it infuse. After four to six weeks, strain out the liquid and bottle it in a dropper bottle. Take two to three droppers full anywhere from thirty minutes to one hour before bedtime. At bedtime, take another two to three droppers full of this formula. If you happen to wake up in the night and find yourself in the same situation where you cannot fall back asleep, take two droppers full again. Before bedtime, avoid looking at blue light from screens to help your brain prepare for sleep. Try doing a relaxing activity, like soaking in a warm bath with Epsom salt. Make it a point to get a good night's sleep and set regular and consistent bedtimes.

INSOMNIA RELIEF TEA

Linden flower is a wonderful alkaline herb for insomnia because it is sedative and calming. It pairs great with California poppy because California poppy is nervine and helps with minor aches and pains as well. Together, these potent flowers create a tea that helps to bring on sleep naturally and ease the body and mind. Combine one teaspoon each of California poppy and linden flower in a tea bag and infuse this in very hot water for five to seven minutes. Drink one to two cups of this tea around one hour prior to bedtime. Unwind with an activity such as meditation or a warm bath after drinking this tea.

SWEET DREAMS TEA

Chamomile and lavender have been utilized for thousands of years to help with sleep issues, as well as anxiety, stress, and nerve issues. They are also gentle enough to be enjoyed by children and adults alike. Chamomile's antispasmodic properties come in handy when helping the body get to sleep. It can also help settle the mind. Lavender helps calm the body and slow things down a bit. It is especially useful if you are frustrated, agitated, or overwhelmed. Combine one teaspoon of chamomile flowers and one teaspoon of lavender buds in a tea bag and infuse this in hot water for five to seven minutes. Drink one to three cups of this tea around one hour before bedtime. Chamomile and lavender also pair well when used in aromatherapy. If you have a diffuser and essential oils, try diffusing five drops of chamomile and five drops of lavender in your room at bedtime to expedite sleep.

ten to twenty drops of essential oils like peppermint, eucalyptus, turmeric, ginger, or copaiba. These help manage inflammation. Pour the ointment into jars to cool. When it cools, it will take on a salve-like consistency that is easy to apply to any area you choose and stays in place. Use this ointment as often as you need for relief from sore muscles, joints, and areas of trauma. As with any salve, avoid getting it in the eyes or mucous membranes.

Menstrual Cycle Irregularities

Remedies

Steady Cycle Tea

By far, one of the best herbs for balancing the hormones and fixing issues that lead to menstrual irregularities is vitex, or chaste tree berry. This berry is an adaptogen, meaning it is a special type of herb that brings balance to whatever is out of balance in the body. It can target the cause and work to bring healing and restoration. Some adaptogenic herbs target the immune system or energy levels in the body, but chaste tree berry targets hormone abnormalities in women specifically. Whether the issue is with high estrogen, progesterone, or prolactin levels, chaste tree berry can help get the levels where they need to be so you can have a normal menstrual cycle.

After taking chaste tree berry for several months steadily, you may begin to notice that your menstrual cycles are right on time and not as painful as they once were. It does need to be taken on a regular basis and for several months before you begin to notice a change.

However, once you begin to notice a difference, you will feel much better emotionally and physically. Drink a tea made with chaste tree berries daily for best results. Infuse one teaspoon of dried chaste tree berries in one cup of very hot water for seven to ten minutes. Add some raw honey to taste, as chaste tree berries can be bitter depending on how potent they are. You may not notice a change right away, but keep drinking this tea and give the berries a chance to change your hormones for the better.

BLEED ON TEA

A menstrual cycle should come each month, optimally every twenty eight days. A regular cycle is a sign of health and hormonal balance. If you start to notice a change in your menstrual cycles, this could be a sign you need to look into your hormone levels. If your cycles are getting farther and farther apart, you might look into drinking the chaste tree berry tea daily (as detailed above). If your cycle still hasn't come and you know for sure you are not pregnant, you can try bringing it one with contribo. This alkaline herb has been utilized for centuries for its emmenagogue properties. Try infusing one teaspoon of contribo into one cup of hot water for ten to fifteen minutes. Drink one cup of this daily until your cycle begins. Begin drinking chaste tree berry tea daily to manage this as well.

DAILY SOOTHING MENSTRUAL TEA

Raspberry Leaf is a nourishing uterine tonic. These leaves can help tone the uterus and keep it healthy. Stinging nettle is a highly nutritious alkaline herb that can provide the body with the nutrients it needs to stay healthy with balanced hormones. When combined in a tea, these two herbs work well for maintaining menstrual and uterine health. Infuse one teaspoon each of dried red raspberry leaf and stinging nettle into one cup of hot water for five to seven minutes before consuming. Drink one cup of this daily for a healthy menstrual cycle.

DYSMENORRHEA TEA

Damiana is an alkaline herb that can help with premenstrual syndrome symptoms like headaches, mood swings, and cramps. Yarrow is known for its ability to staunch heavy blood flow in menstruating women who have issues with losing too much blood and tissue. If you have issues with heavy, painful cycles or premenstrual syndrome, this tea can help.

Infuse one teaspoon each of dried yarrow leaves and flowers, as well as damiana leaves, into one cup of hot water. Let this infuse for seven to ten minutes to make a stronger tea. Drink one to three cups of this daily throughout your menstrual cycle to manage symptoms. You may also drink this tea the week before your menstrual cycle to manage premenstrual syndrome symptoms.

CRAMP RELIEF TEA

Some women experience painful cramping during their cycles. Cramping is normal to an extent, but painful cramping that leads to nausea and diarrhea each month is not normal. This could be a sign that something else is going on in the body. If you find yourself experiencing these symptoms each month, consider starting a daily regimen of chaste tree berry tea. To further help manage symptoms during your cycle; try a tea made with cramp bark and valerian. Both have analgesic properties, but cramp bark is specifically known for helping with uterine cramps. It is anti-spasmodic and soothes muscles. Valerian is a sedative and has analgesic properties that can help manage cramps. Combine one teaspoon of dried and chopped valerian root with one teaspoon of cramp bark in a tea bag. Let this infuse in very hot water for ten to fifteen minutes before consuming. Drink one to three cups of this as needed when you are experiencing debilitating cramps. The valerian may make you sleepy, but this is a good thing because rest can help you recover faster.

NAUSEA AND VOMITING

REMEDIES

CALMING TEA

Chamomile and nettle can work together in a tea for calming the nerves, as well as nausea that may be interfering with your life. Chamomile's aroma is enough for some people to quell nausea. It is anti-spasmodic and helps settle spasms that lead to vomiting. Nettle can help replace lost nutrients if you have been vomiting. Combine one teaspoon of dried chamomile flowers and one teaspoon of dried stinging nettle leaves in a tea bag and infuse this in hot water for seven to ten minutes. Add a small amount of raw honey to taste. Drink one to three cups of this tea as needed to manage nausea and vomiting, as well as to calm the body and ease stress.

Ginger Emergency Formula

Ginger is an excellent herb for reducing nausea and vomiting. Just the scent alone can help stave off nausea. Ginger can settle an upset stomach and reduce gastrointestinal discomfort. Combining ginger with peppermint is one of the best known remedies for managing nausea. Peppermint is naturally carminative and helps ease digestive woes. Its light, invigorating scent is uplifting and can eliminate nausea. Peppermint blends well with ginger both aromatically and in formulas for nausea. Try combining one part peppermint leaves and one part chopped ginger root in a glass jar. Pour alcohol over the plant material, covering it at least three-fourths of the way. Top the rest off with raw honey. Shake the bottle well to help it blend. Store this somewhere in a cool, dark place to infuse for four to six weeks. After four to six weeks are up, strain out the liquid through a strainer and bottle it. Take five milliliters of this formula as needed to eradicate nausea, an upset stomach, gas, bloating, and other digestive discomforts.

RASH

REMEDIES

Dry Rash Salve

For rashes that are inflamed, red, irritated, and dry, try a soothing salve made with chickweed. Chickweed is one of the most effective herbs for calming the skin. It provides a cooling sensation that helps to lessen irritation and provide relief. The addition of calendula flowers makes this salve extra effective and healing. Calendula is known for its skin-healing properties. It is soothing, healing, and regenerating. Infuse one part chickweed and one part calendula in a carrier oil (jojoba is good for this type of rash). Let this sit in a cool, dark place for four to six weeks to infuse, or you can infuse faster with heat. If you want to make this rash salve faster, you can put your plants in the carrier oil like normal and then place the jar of oil and plants (make sure its glass) in a pan of hot water on the stove for up to twelve hours. Make sure the heat is not turned up to high; this is best infused under low heat for an extended period of time. After the plant material has successfully infused, strain out the oil. In a double boiler, add eight ounces of chickweed and calendula-infused oil and one ounce of beeswax. Let this sit under low heat in the double boiler until the beeswax has completely melted. Stir the beeswax and oil together well. If you wish, you may add ten to fifteen drops of lavender essential oil (or any other skin-soothing oil) to the mixture. Pour this into jars to cool and it will take on a thicker, salve-like consistency. This salve is perfect for application on the skin because it is not runny. It stays in place so it can heal the area faster. Apply it as often as needed to rashes.

Weepy Rash Poultice

Weepy rashes are often the result of contact with something that causes a reaction. For example, poisonous plants like poison ivy are known to cause a weepy rash that itches fiercely. For these rashes, you will need a plant that is soothing, healing, and promotes drying of the rash. One of the most popular plants for treating weepy rashes is jewelweed. It is a very common plant found along creeks and wet areas throughout North America. It is often found growing in abundance in the summertime. It is distinguished by its "jewel-like" red and orange flowers hanging from the plant like a necklace. Legend has it that jewelweed grows where poison ivy grows because nature knows what we need to heal. The inner stems have a gel-like substance that is somewhat reminiscent to aloe vera. It makes the perfect poultice because of this. Mash up jewelweed stems until you have a nice poultice. Apply this directly to the affected area as often as needed to treat a weepy rash. Harvest enough jewelweed to make multiple poultices so you can keep treating the rash until it heals.

Skin-Soothing Tea

Treat skin from the inside out with a tea that promotes healthy skin. One of the most popular plants for beautiful skin is rose. This is because it is gently astringent and emollient. Rose is also wonderful in tea and can be consumed to promote healthy skin. In addition to rose, hibiscus flowers have been used traditionally to treat skin issues. Hibiscus is also hydrating to dull skin, giving it a glow and vibrancy. Hibiscus and rose combine perfectly in a tea for skin health. Combine one teaspoon of dried rose petals with one teaspoon of dried hibiscus flower and infuse this into one cup of hot water for five to seven minutes. Tea made from these flowers will turn a gorgeous pink color. Drink one to two cups a day to promote healthy skin. It is said that beauty begets beauty, so it is no wonder such beautiful flowers make the skin beautiful.

Rash Wash

For a calming wash to treat a variety of rashes, try a wash made with chickweed, chamomile, and witch hazel. Chickweed works to treat inflammation and irritation, chamomile works to reduce redness and heal angry skin, and witch hazel's astringent properties work to tighten, tone, and heal skin tissue. Together, these three powerful herbs can cleanse and heal a rash fast. Start by boiling two cups of water on the stove. Fill a glass jar with one teaspoon each of chickweed, chamomile, and witch hazel bark. Carefully pour the water over the plant material in the jar and let this infuse for one to two hours. When it has completely cooled, wash the affected areas with this liquid thoroughly. You can also soak a clean cloth in this to apply to the rash to further promote healing after you wash the area well. Refrigerate what you don't use. This will keep in the refrigerator for up to three days, so make sure you use it up within this time period, treating the rash often.

Sinusitis/Stuffy Nose

Remedies

Sinus-Clearing Steam Bath

A steamy bath is a very effective way to break up stubborn mucous in the sinuses and reduce congestion. The addition of eucalyptus leaves can help release oils that further work to open the airways and prevent infection in the sinus area. Treat yourself to a soothing eucalyptus bath by running hot water (as hot as you can stand). Shut the curtain or door to trap in steam. Place one half cup of dried and crumbled eucalyptus leaves in a muslin bag. Shut the bag well and place it in the bath water to soak and infuse. Get in the bath and soak as long as you can, practicing deep breathing techniques to better inhale the healing eucalyptus steam. Do this as needed to treat and prevent sinus issues.

Sinus-Relieving Tea

For a tea to treat sinus infections and mucous in the sinus area, try utilizing a combination of sage and pau d' arco bark. Sage is an expectorant and can help to get mucous out of the body. It is also antimicrobial, so it can help treat any infection in the sinuses. Pau d' arco is is highly antimicrobial and has antibiotic properties that work to target any infection before it causes problems in the body. Together, sage and pau d' arco can effectively treat and prevent sinus infections. When the sinuses are congested, the trapped mucous in the sinus cavities can begin to grow bacteria that leads to infection. Fevers, chills, and serious headaches in the sinus area can develop as a result. This tea can help take care of these issues before they get serious. Infuse one teaspoon each of pau d' arco bark and sage leaves into one cup of hot water for seven to ten minutes. Drink one to two cups daily to release trapped mucous and kill infection-causing germs in the sinuses.

Mucous-Freeing Tea

To break up mucous, try a combination of mullein and pleurisy root. Mullein is a known herbal demulcent and expectorant. Pleurisy root is also expectorant and is used to target mucous and fluid in the airways. Pleurisy root is a very common "weed" found throughout North America. It often goes by the name "butterfly weed" because butterflies love this pollinator. It has bright red-orange flowers that bloom in the summer. The root of this plant is what is used medicinally, so make sure if you harvest any to leave some as well. Combine one teaspoon of dried and chopped mullein leaves with one teaspoon of dried and chopped pleurisy root in a tea bag. Infuse this into a cup of very hot water for seven to ten minutes before consuming. Drink one to three cups daily to release mucous and fluid in the sinuses, bronchial area, and lungs.

Sore Throat

Remedies

Sore Throat Tea

Wild Bergamot, or "bee balm" as it is sometimes called, was used extensively by indigenous people in North America to treat a sore throat. This powerful plant was introduced to settlers who were astounded at its effectiveness. Studies show wild bergamot to be highly antimicrobial and potent. It has a chemical profile similar to thyme. Another native North American plant that was used in conjunction with wild bergamot is Echinacea. There are several medicinal species of Echinacea throughout North America, but one of the most studied species is *Echinacea purpurea.* Echinacea has been shown in multiple studies to have antiviral, antiseptic, and anti-inflammatory properties. It has been used for everything from a sore throat to boosting the immune system to prevent sickness. Combining wild bergamot with Echinacea will help boost the immune system to fight off any germs responsible for the sore throat. Combine one teaspoon of dried and chopped Echinacea (all parts of the plant are used) and one teaspoon of dried and chopped wild bergamot aerial parts. Infuse this in a cup of hot water for seven to ten minutes. Consume one to three cups daily to treat a sore throat, strep throat, or any other throat infection.

Herbal Gargle

Pau d' arco is one of the best alkaline plants for treating a sore throat caused by the streptococcus infection. Its strong antibiotic properties target the bacteria and kill it, restoring health and bringing relief. The addition of herbs like sage and yarrow help to cleanse, soothe, and heal affected tissues in the throat. To make a gargle with these plants, start by bringing one cup of water to boil on the stove. Add one teaspoon each of pau d' arco, sage, and yarrow. Bring the heat down and let these infuse for fifteen minutes. Add a teaspoon of sea salt or Himalayan salt and let this dissolve well. Strain out the liquid and let it cool completely. Measure out one half ounce of this liquid and gargle it for one to two minutes, making sure to get the liquid to the back of the throat as you gargle. Spit this out and repeat up to five times daily to treat a throat infection. Drink the "Sore Throat Tea" detailed above for even faster healing.

THROAT-SOOTHING TEA

Sometimes a sore throat can feel extremely uncomfortable and make it hard to swallow. This affects eating and drinking, leading to poor health and dehydration. If you find that you have a sore throat that makes it difficult to swallow, try a combination of chamomile and chaparral for relief. Chamomile calms the surface tissue as much as it calms the mind. It can soothe the area, while reducing inflammation. Chaparral is highly anti-inflammatory, helping to bring down inflammation in the throat that leads to pain and discomfort. Combine one teaspoon each of chaparral and chamomile in a tea bag and infuse this in hot water for five to seven minutes. Add one to three teaspoons of raw honey to help further soothe the throat, as well as kill bacteria that may be causing the sore throat. Drink one to two cups daily for soothing relief.

FRUITY GARGLE

Elderberry isn't just great for treating a virus and boosting the immune system. It is also a powerfully anti-inflammatory fruit. It can relieve a sore throat effectively, while also reducing any drainage that may be causing irritation in the throat. Red raspberry leaf is a mild astringent and can help tighten and tone the throat tissues, relieving soreness and pain. Its astringent properties are the result of tannins in the leaves. Herbs with tannins have traditionally been used to treat inflamed tissues both internally and externally. A combination of elderberry and red raspberry leaves make a fruity and delicious way to treat a sore throat! To make this gargle, start by boiling two cups of water on the stove. Add one tablespoon each of dried and crumbled red raspberry leaves and dried elderberries. Lower the heat and let this simmer until the liquid is reduced by half. You should have one cup of liquid when you are finished. Strain out the liquid and add two tablespoons of raw honey. Stir it in well until it is completely dissolved. Let the gargle cool completely before use. Gargle one half ounce of this liquid for two minutes as needed for relief from a sore throat. Refrigerate the gargle and continue using it as needed until it is gone.

Sweet Cough Drops

Does a nasty cough and congestion have your throat sore and inflamed? Too much coughing can really irritate the throat tissues, resulting in tenderness and pain. Ginger and sage combine in this remedy to bring relief fast. For a soothing, antitussive treatment, start by boiling two cups of water on the stove. Add two tablespoons each of dried and chopped ginger and sage. Reduce heat and let this simmer until the liquid is reduced by half. Carefully strain out the liquid and clean out the pot. Add the herb-infused liquid back to the pot under medium heat. Add one to one-and-a-half cups of raw honey and stir everything until it is well-blended. Bring this back to a boil and keep it boiling until the honey and water mixture begins to thicken. When you are able to take small amounts on a spoon and place them on wax paper and they do not run, but rather harden, this is when you know it is ready. Be very careful because this honey mixture is very hot and can burn the skin easily. Keep taking small spoonful's of the mixture and dropping them onto the wax paper. Leave them to harden fully. You can speed up this process by putting your sheets of wax paper in the refrigerator for several hours. When they are fully hard, sprinkle them with powdered cinnamon, ginger, or turmeric to add additional medicinal power while preventing them from sticking together in a container. Take these tasty drops as needed to help with a cough or sore throat.

SPRAINS AND STRAINS

REMEDIES

SOFT TISSUE INJURY LINIMENT

For sprains, one of the best herbs to reduce inflammation and tighten stretched ligaments and/or tendons is Solomon's seal. This native North American plant has been used traditionally for inflammation and trauma. It almost works like an adaptogenic herb with its ability to tighten or loosen, depending on what the body needs. The root of this plant is used in herbal remedies, both externally and internally. Always harvest this plant mindfully, as it is not common in some areas. Harvest the roots, clean them, and chop them well. Lay them to dry. When they are completely dry, fill a clean glass jar with the root pieces. Cover them completely in a carrier oil. Let this sit and infuse for four to six weeks in a cool, dark place. Strain out the oil and add eight ounces of it to a double boiler. Next, add one ounce of beeswax pellets. Heat this gently until the beeswax melts, making sure to stir continually. Pour this into small jars to cool. Apply a liberal amount as needed to injured joints or areas of the body that have sustained trauma.

TOPICAL PAIN RELIEF

Arnica is a flower known for its ability to ease pain, especially when it comes to pain from injured joints. Historically, it has been a major ingredient in an oil infusion called "trauma oil." Trauma oil is created using several different plants in addition to arnica. These include St. John's Wort, known for helping nerve pain and inflammation, and calendula flowers, known for soothing and calming. Infusing all three of these flowers in olive oil creates a powerful topical pain relief remedy. Fill a jar with one part calendula, one part arnica, and one part St. John's Wort flowers. If possible, it is best to use fresh or wilted St. John's Wort flowers. Cover the flowers completely with a good quality olive oil and let this infuse for four to six weeks before straining it out. Shake your jar daily to help the flowers infuse better. Strain out the oil and bottle it in a tinted jar to keep sunlight from degrading it. Label it and store it in a cool, dark place to use as needed. Apply a liberal amount to affected areas as often as you can to promote healing, lower inflammation, and reduce pain. Any time you are working with arnica, be sure to keep it out of open wounds. This includes cuts and scrapes. Arnica is fine for the skin and very effective at what it does, but it should not get into the bloodstream or it could cause issues.

Quick-Acting Pain Relief

For quick pain relief from the swelling and trauma associated with sprains and related injuries, try a twofold approach: First, apply a large cabbage leaf to the affected area. Cabbage leaves work quickly to lower inflammation and reduce pain. You may remove and reapply a new leaf as needed. Next, take two droppers-full of a tincture made with white willow bark. Repeat this every two to three hours as needed for pain. White willow contains a compound called salicin that specifically targets pain and inflammation in the body. This compound is still used today to create over-the-counter pain relievers like aspirin. However, taking white willow tincture doesn't affect the kidneys or gut like aspirin. To create this tincture, shave off the inner bark of the white willow tree. Fill a jar with shavings and completely cover them in at least 80 proof alcohol. Let this infuse for four to six weeks and then strain out the liquid. Store your tincture in a cool, dark place to use for pain relief.

Sweet Relief Tea

A tea made with chamomile and linden flowers can help provide relief from pain, while promoting relaxation and reducing any stress related to pain. Combine one teaspoon of linden flowers with one teaspoon of chamomile flowers in a tea bag and infuse this in one cup of hot water for five to seven minutes. Add a small amount of raw honey to taste and enjoy a cup of this soothing tea up to three times daily for relief from pain from sprains, muscle aches, joint aches, and even headaches.

STRESS

REMEDIES

RESCUE ELIXIR

For an elixir that comes to the rescue to calm the body and mind, blue vervain is a true friend. Blue vervain calms the nerves and promotes relaxation quickly. Create a strong but sweet extract with blue vervain by filling a jar with the aerial parts of the plant. Cover them three-fourths of the way with at least 80 proof alcohol and the rest of the way with raw honey or brandy. Shake this well each day and store it in a cool, dark place to infuse. After four to six weeks, strain out your elixir and take two to three droppers full when you are feeling overwhelmed, stressed, or anxious. Do this up to three times daily.

SOOTHE UP TEA

Always there to help soothe the body and provide relief, linden flowers can be an ally for stress and stress-related issues. If you find yourself in need of some serious soothing, try infusing one teaspoon of linden flowers into one cup of hot water for five to seven minutes. Add raw honey to taste. Drink one to five cups of this tasty tea daily for management of stress.

NERVE SOOTHING TEA

For herbs that work specifically on the nerves, try a tea made with skullcap and valerian root. Skullcap is a wonderful herb for combating frustration, anxiousness, and the feeling of being "on-edge." Valerian is a powerful nervine that helps to relax the nerves, muscles, and mind. Combining these two nervine herbs is sure to soothe aggravated nerves. Start by adding one teaspoon each of dried skullcap (aerial parts) and dried and chopped valerian root to a tea bag. Infuse this into one cup of very hot water for seven to ten minutes. Drink one to three cups as needed to soothe the nerves and find relief.

CALMING TEA

Lavender and lupulo can help calm you down when you need it most. Lavender boasts the ability to calm the body and has even been shown in studies to lower blood pressure. This is an important attribute since stress and anxiety almost always raise blood pressure. Lupulo, or hops, is a nervine and sedative plant that help quiet a racing mind and relax the body. Combine one teaspoon of dried lavender buds and one teaspoon of hops in a tea bag and infuse this in a cup of hot water for five to ten minutes. (Let it sit for the full ten minutes for a stronger tea). Drink one to three cups of this tea daily to manage stress and help pacify the body so it can stay healthy and function properly.

SHAKE-IT-OFF TEA

Chamomile has been associated with stress relief for centuries, and it is still used today to help reduce stress and anxiety. Motherwort is a gentle and helpful herb for stress as well. It is also great for heart health and lowering blood pressure. It can provide quick relief from tension and nervous conditions. Both chamomile and motherwort complement each other and taste great together in a tea for stress. Combine one teaspoon each of chamomile flowers and motherwort (aerial parts) in a tea bag. Let this infuse in one cup of hot water for seven to ten minutes before enjoying. Try drinking one to two cups for times when you feel overwhelmed or nervous.

WEIGHT LOSS AND BELLY FAT

REMEDIES

Detox and Cleanse using Alkaline herbs
Build muscles
Take protein from plant sources
Limit Starches
Exercise and fasting
Perform Coffee scrub
Lots of hot teas.

WOUNDS

REMEDIES

WOUND WASH

The first step for wound care is to wash a wound well. This may very well be one of the most important things you can do to treat a wound correctly. Yarrow makes an excellent wound wash because of its strong antiseptic properties. It is also helps promote healing for the wound. Make a simple wound wash with the aerial parts of the yarrow plant by infusing two teaspoons of dried yarrow in one cup of hot water for fifteen to twenty minutes. When this has completely cooled, strain it out and wash the wound with it. Repeat this prior to treating with a salve or ointment as often as possible to help a wound heal fast. Consider applying raw honey to the wound after washing it with yarrow because the honey can help kill dangerous bacteria and promote recovery.

PINE RESIN SALVE

Pine resin is another great wound remedy because it contains antimicrobial properties that help cleanse and heal a wound. The prevention of infection is key to getting a wound to heal properly, and pine resin is perfect for this task.

Pine trees have been used medicinally for generations because many parts of the tree benefit humans. For example, the needles have been used traditionally to treat scurvy and are a good source of vitamin C. The needles are also steam distilled into an essential oil to help open the airways and promote respiratory health. The resin is the substance the tree produces when it has a wound. The tree tries to "heal" its own wound by covering the area with this sticky substance. Pine resin can be collected from the pine three where there is a missing limb or abrasion. Only if completely necessary should you drill a small hole to collect the resin. Visit your pine trees daily to collect resin until you have at least one tablespoon. You may need a knife or object to scrape the sap from the tree if it has ran down the trunk. In a double boiler, add the pine resin to eight ounces of a healing carrier oil like olive oil or emu oil. Let this melt together gently until the pine resin is no longer in chunks. Add one ounce of beeswax and allow this to melt into the oil. Stir under low heat until everything is blended together sufficiently. Remove the mixture from heat. At this time, you may consider adding ten to twenty drops of a wound-healing essential oil like tea tree or lavender. Pour the salve into jars to cool. Apply to wounds after washing them to promote restoration of any skin trauma.

TOPICAL APPLICATION FOR ABRASIONS

Yarrow and chickweed work perfectly in a salve to target several issues related to wound healing. For starters, yarrow prevents infection and stops bleeding. Chickweed comes to the rescue for angry, irritated skin that has been agitated by a wound. It works to cool and soothe the skin while repairing any damage. Infuse one part chickweed (wilted or dried) and one part yarrow in a carrier oil for four to six weeks, shaking it daily. Keep your herb infusion in a cool, dark place during this time. Strain out the oil after four to six weeks. You may choose to treat abrasions by using this oil alone or combining eight ounces of the oil with one ounce of beeswax in a double boiler for a salve that has a thicker consistency. Apply this to abrasions as needed (after washing) to mend the skin and keep bacteria at bay.

TOPICAL WASH FOR CUTS

For cuts, especially ones that seem to have a hard time with blood clotting, try a wash made with yarrow and shepherd's purse. This wash works to cleanse a wound, stop bleeding, and repair the broken skin. Infuse two teaspoons each of dried yarrow and shepherd's purse into one cup of hot water for fifteen to twenty minutes. Strain out the liquid and allow it to cool completely. Apply a liberal amount of this wash to cuts and minor lacerations prior to treatment with a salve or raw honey. You can also soak a small clean rag in this wash and apply it to a cut for several minutes to speed up healing and aid in skin renewal.

BONUS RECIPES

1. ROASTED OKRA WITH HABANERO

SERVING: 2

Preparation time: 5 minutes; Cook time: 12 minutes;
Nutritional Info: 76 Cal; 2 g Fats; 2 g Protein; 6 g Carb; 2 g Fiber;

INGREDIENTS

- ½ pound okra, ends trimmed
- 2 habanero peppers, sliced
- 2 teaspoons avocado oil
- ½ teaspoon salt
- 1/3 teaspoon ground thyme

Extra:
- 1 tablespoon key lime juice

DIRECTIONS

- Plug in an air fryer, place the fryer basket in it, grease it with cooking oil, shut the air fryer with its lid, set the temperature to 350 degrees F, and let it preheat.
- Meanwhile, cut the okra into slices, place them in a medium bowl, add remaining ingredients, and then toss until coated.
- Arrange the prepared okra and habanero mixture in the air fryer, shut with its lid, and then cook for 12 minutes, tossing halfway.
- Serve straight away.

2. ROASTED OKRA WITH TOMATOES

SERVING: 2

Preparation time: 5 minutes; Cook time: 12 minutes;
Nutritional Info: 88 Cal; 4 g Fats; 4 g Protein; 11 g Carb; 4 g Fiber;

INGREDIENTS

- ½ pound okra, ends trimmed
- 4 cherry tomatoes, chopped
- ½ of medium red bell pepper, chopped
- 2 teaspoons avocado oil

- 1/3 teaspoon dried thyme

Extra:
- ½ teaspoon salt
- 1 tablespoon key lime juice

DIRECTIONS

- Plug in an air fryer, place the fryer basket in it, grease it with cooking oil, shut the air fryer with its lid, set the temperature to 350 degrees F, and let it preheat.
- Meanwhile, cut the okra into slices, place them in a medium bowl, add remaining ingredients, and then toss until coated.
- Arrange the prepared okra and tomato mixture in the air fryer, shut with its lid, and then cook for 12 minutes, tossing halfway.
- Serve straight away.

3. MUSHROOMS STUFFED AVOCADOS

SERVING: 2

Preparation time: 5 minutes; Cook time: 15 minutes;
Nutritional Info: 73 Cal; 3 g Fats; 5 g Protein; 7 g Carb; 2 g Fiber;

INGREDIENTS

- 1 large avocado, peeled, pitted, halved
- ½ cup chopped mushrooms
- ½ tablespoon chopped basil
- ¼ teaspoon cayenne pepper
- ¼ cup shredded Brazil nut cheese

Extra:
- ¼ teaspoon salt

DIRECTIONS

- Plug in an air fryer, place the fryer basket in it, grease it with cooking oil, shut the air fryer with its lid, set the temperature to 400 degrees F, and let it preheat.
- Meanwhile, prepare the avocado and for this, cut the avocado in half, season with salt and cayenne pepper.
- Arrange the prepared avocado halves in the air fryer in a single layer, shut with its lid, and then cook for 12 minutes.

- Then stuff the avocado with mushrooms, sprinkle cheese on top, sprinkle with basil, and continue air frying the avocado halves for 3 to 5 minutes until done.
- Serve straight away.

4. ROASTED OKRA WITH LIME AND DILL

SERVING: 2

Preparation time: 5 minutes; Cook time: 12 minutes;
Nutritional Info: 65.1 Cal; 3.7 g Fats; 3.7 g Protein; 7.3 g Carb; 3.2 g Fiber;

INGREDIENTS

- ½ pound okra, ends trimmed
- 1/3 teaspoon dried dill
- 1 tablespoon vinegar
- ½ tablespoon chopped basil
- ½ of key lime, juiced

Extra:
- 2 teaspoons sesame seeds oil

DIRECTIONS

- Plug in an air fryer, place the fryer basket in it, grease it with cooking oil, shut the air fryer with its lid, set the temperature to 350 degrees F, and let it preheat.
- Meanwhile, cut the okra into slices, place them in a medium bowl, add remaining ingredients, and then toss until coated.
- Arrange the prepared okra slices in the air fryer in a single layer, shut with its lid, and then cook for 12 minutes, tossing halfway.
- Serve straight away.

5. AVOCADO AND SQUASH

SERVING: 2

Preparation time: 5 minutes; Cook time: 12 minutes;
Nutritional Info: 115 Cal; 0.3 g Fats; 2.3 g Protein; 29.9 g Carb; 9 g Fiber;

INGREDIENTS

- 1 avocado, peeled, pitted, chopped
- 1 medium butternut squash, peeled, cored, chopped

- ¼ teaspoon cayenne pepper
- ¼ teaspoon dried thyme
- ¼ teaspoon chopped basil

Extra:
- 1 tablespoon sesame seeds oil
- ½ teaspoon salt

DIRECTIONS

- Plug in an air fryer, place the fryer basket in it, grease it with cooking oil, shut the air fryer with its lid, set the temperature to 350 degrees F, and let it preheat.
- Meanwhile, take a large bowl, place all the ingredients in it and then stir until combined.
- Add prepared vegetables in the air fryer, shut with its lid, and then cook for 12 minutes, turning halfway.
- Serve straight away.

6. OKRA WITH ONION AND TOMATO

SERVING: 2

Preparation time: 5 minutes; Cook time: 12 minutes;
Nutritional Info: 50 Cal; 0.6 g Fats; 2.8 g Protein; 10.7 g Carb; 3 g Fiber;

INGREDIENTS

- ½ pound okra, ends trimmed
- 1 medium white onion, peeled, sliced
- 2 teaspoons sesame seeds oil
- 1 medium tomato, chopped
- ½ teaspoon dried thyme

Extra:
- ½ teaspoon salt
- 1/3 teaspoon cayenne pepper

DIRECTIONS

- Plug in an air fryer, place the fryer basket in it, grease it with cooking oil, shut the air fryer with its lid, set the temperature to 350 degrees F, and let it preheat.
- Meanwhile, cut the okra into slices, place them in a medium bowl, add onion slices, tomatoes, salt, cayenne pepper, thyme, and oil, and then toss until coated.

- Arrange the prepared okra and onion in the air fryer in a single layer, shut with its lid, and then cook for 12 minutes, tossing halfway.
- Serve straight away.

7. AVOCADO LETTUCE WRAP

SERVING: 2

Preparation time: 5 minutes; Cook time: 10 minutes;
Nutritional Info: 157 Cal; 8 g Fats; 2 g Protein; 12.5 g Carb; 2 g Fiber;

INGREDIENTS

- 1 avocado, peeled, pitted, diced
- ½ teaspoon cayenne pepper
- ¼ teaspoon dried thyme
- 2 large lettuce leaves
- 1 key lime, juiced

Extra:
- ½ teaspoon salt
- 1 teaspoon sesame seeds oil

DIRECTIONS

- Plug in an air fryer, place the fryer basket in it, grease it with cooking oil, shut the air fryer with its lid, set the temperature to 400 degrees F, and let it preheat.
- Meanwhile, take a medium bowl, place the avocado in it, add salt, cayenne pepper, thyme, and oil, and then stir until mixed.
- Place avocado in the air fryer in a single layer, shut with its lid, and then cook for 10 minutes, tossing halfway.
- When done, divide avocado between the lettuce leaves, drizzle with lime juice and then serve.

8. PEPPER AND LETTUCE WRAP

SERVING: 2

Preparation time: 5 minutes; Cook time: 10 minutes;
Nutritional Info: 48 Cal; 0.3 g Fats; 1.6 g Protein; 9.5 g Carb; 2.3 g Fiber;

INGREDIENTS

- 3 medium red bell peppers, cored, diced

- 1/4 teaspoon salt
- ¼ teaspoon cayenne pepper
- 2 tablespoons key lime juice
- 2 large leaves of lettuce

Extra:
-

DIRECTIONS

- Plug in an air fryer, place the fryer basket in it, grease it with cooking oil, shut the air fryer with its lid, set the temperature to 400 degrees F, and let it preheat.
- Meanwhile, prepare the peppers and for this, take a large bowl, place peppers in it, add salt, cayenne pepper, and lime juice and then toss until coated.
- Arrange the prepared bell peppers in the air fryer in a single layer, spray oil on top, shut with its lid, and then cook for 8 to 10 minutes until golden brown, turning halfway.
- Divide the bell peppers evenly between two lettuce leaves, wrap the leaves and then serve.

9. SQUASH WITH SAGE

SERVING: 2

Preparation time: 5 minutes; Cook time: 12 minutes;
Nutritional Info: 90 Cal; 4 g Fats; 1 g Protein; 13 g Carb; 4 g Fiber;

INGREDIENTS

- 2 butternut squashes, peeled, cored, diced
- ¼ teaspoon dried sage
- 1/3 teaspoon dried thyme
- 1/3 teaspoon dried oregano
- 2 tablespoons sesame seeds oil

Extra:
- ¾ teaspoon salt
- 1/3 teaspoon cayenne pepper
- 2 key limes, juiced

DIRECTIONS

- Plug in an air fryer, place the fryer basket in it, grease it with cooking oil, shut the air fryer with its lid, set the temperature to 400 degrees F, and let it preheat.
- Meanwhile, take a large bowl, place all the ingredients in it and then toss until well coated.
- Arrange the prepared squash pieces in the air fryer in a single layer, spray oil on top, shut with its lid, and then cook for 12 minutes until golden brown, turning halfway.
- Serve straight away.

10. PEPPERS STUFFED MUSHROOMS

SERVING: 2

Preparation time: 5 minutes; Cook time: 10 minutes;
Nutritional Info: 148 Cal; 8.5 g Fats; 7 g Protein; 12 g Carb; 2 g Fiber;

INGREDIENTS

- 4 whole button mushrooms, destemmed
- ½ teaspoon cayenne pepper
- ½ cup chopped red bell pepper
- ½ cup chopped green bell pepper
- ¼ teaspoon ground coriander

Extra:

- ½ teaspoon salt
- ¼ teaspoon dried thyme
- 2 tablespoons sesame seeds oil
- 4 tablespoons hazel nut cheese

DIRECTIONS

- Plug in an air fryer, place the fryer basket in it, grease it with cooking oil, shut the air fryer with its lid, set the temperature to 350 degrees F, and let it preheat.
- Meanwhile, prepare the mushrooms and for this, take a small bowl, place oil in it, add salt, cayenne pepper, and coriander, stir until combined, and then brush this mixture all over the mushrooms.
- Arrange the prepared mushrooms in the air fryer in a single layer, shut with its lid, and then cook for 10 minutes until golden brown, turning halfway.
- Take a medium bowl, place chopped peppers in it and then stir until mixed.

- Stuffed the mushrooms with bell peppers, sprinkle cheese and thyme on top and then continue air frying for 2 minutes until the cheese has melted.
- Serve straight away.

11. TOMATO AND ONION STUFFED ZUCCHINI

SERVING: 2

Preparation time: 5 minutes; Cook time: 20 minutes;
Nutritional Info: 121 Cal; 3.2 g Fats; 6.2 g Protein; 17 g Carb; 3.5 g Fiber;

INGREDIENTS

- 2 zucchinis, cut in half lengthwise
- ½ cup chopped tomatoes
- ½ cup chopped white onion
- ¼ teaspoon cayenne pepper
- ¼ teaspoon dried thyme

Extra:
- 1 ½ teaspoon salt

DIRECTIONS

- Plug in an air fryer, place the fryer basket in it, grease it with cooking oil, shut the air fryer with its lid, set the temperature to 350 degrees F, and let it preheat.
- Meanwhile, prepare the zucchinis and for this, cut them in half lengthwise, create a well by scooping some center and then sprinkle with 1 teaspoon salt.
- Arrange the prepared zucchinis in the air fryer in a single layer, shut with its lid, and then cook for 20 minutes.
- Take a medium bowl, place tomatoes in it, add remaining ingredients, and stir until combined.
- Spoon the tomato-onion mixture into the zucchini and then serve.

12. MUSHROOMS STUFFED WITH ONION AND TOMATOES

SERVING: 2

Preparation time: 5 minutes; Cook time: 10 minutes;
Nutritional Info: 79.2 Cal; 0.3 g Fats; 3.2 g Protein; 15 g Carb; 2.5 g Fiber;

INGREDIENTS

- 4 whole button mushrooms, destemmed
- ½ cup chopped tomatoes
- ¼ cup chopped white onion
- 2/3 teaspoon Italian seasoning
- 2/3 teaspoon salt

Extra:
- 1 tablespoon avocado oil
- 1 key lime, juiced

DIRECTIONS

- Plug in an air fryer, place the fryer basket in it, grease it with cooking oil, shut the air fryer with its lid, set the temperature to 350 degrees F, and let it preheat.
- Meanwhile, prepare the mushrooms and for this, take a small bowl, place oil in it, add salt and Italian seasoning, stir until combined, and then brush this mixture all over the mushrooms.
- Arrange the prepared mushrooms in the air fryer in a single layer, shut with its lid, and then cook for 10 minutes until golden brown, turning halfway.
- Meanwhile, take a medium bowl, place onion and tomatoes in it, drizzle with lime juice and then stir until mixed.
- When done, let the mushrooms stuffed with the onion-tomato mixture and then serve.

13. ZUCCHINI NOODLES WITH TOMATOES

SERVING: 2

Preparation time: 5 minutes; Cook time: 20 minutes;
Nutritional Info: 154 Cal; 3 g Fats; 4 g Protein; 29 g Carb; 8 g Fiber;

INGREDIENTS

- 2 zucchinis, spiralized into noodles
- 1 cup cherry tomato halves
- ½ teaspoon salt
- 1 key lime, juiced
- 1 tablespoon avocado oil

Extra:
- ½ teaspoon dried thyme
- ¼ teaspoon dried oregano

DIRECTIONS

- Plug in an air fryer, place the fryer basket in it, grease it with cooking oil, shut the air fryer with its lid, set the temperature to 400 degrees F, and let it preheat.
- Meanwhile, take a large bowl, place tomatoes in it, add oil, salt, thyme, and oregano and then toss until well coated.
- Arrange the prepared tomato halves in the air fryer in a single layer, shut with its lid, and then cook for 15 minutes until roasted, turning halfway.
- When done, transfer tomatoes to a bowl, add zucchini noodles and remaining ingredients, and then toss until mixed.
- Take a baking pan greased with oil, spoon zucchini noodles mixture in it, place the pan in the air fryer and cook for 5 minutes until thoroughly hot.
- Serve straight away.

14. OKRA LETTUCE WRAP

SERVING: 2

Preparation time: 5 minutes; Cook time: 10 minutes;
Nutritional Info: 121 Cal; 5.6 g Fats; 6.8 g Protein; 10 g Carb; 1.6 g Fiber;

INGREDIENTS

- ½ pound okra, ends trimmed
- 2 teaspoons avocado oil
- ½ teaspoon salt
- 1/3 teaspoon cayenne pepper
- 2 leaves of lettuce

DIRECTIONS

- Plug in an air fryer, place the fryer basket in it, grease it with cooking oil, shut the air fryer with its lid, set the temperature to 350 degrees F, and let it preheat.
- Meanwhile, cut the okra into slices, place them in a medium bowl, add salt, cayenne pepper, and oil and then toss until coated.
- Arrange the prepared okra slices in the air fryer in a single layer, shut with its lid, and then cook for 12 minutes, tossing halfway.
- When done, divide okra evenly between lettuce leaves, wrap and then serve.

15. BELL PEPPER STUFFED WITH WILD RICE

SERVING: 2

Preparation time: 10 minutes; Cook time: 20 minutes;
Nutritional Info: 106 Cal; 4 g Fats; 2 g Protein; 10 g Carb; 2 g Fiber;

INGREDIENTS

- 2 medium red bell peppers, cored
- 2 cherry tomatoes, chopped
- 1 cup cooked wild rice
- 1 teaspoon dried oregano
- 2 tablespoons hazel nut cheese
- ½ teaspoon onion powder
- ½ teaspoon salt

DIRECTIONS

- Plug in an air fryer, place the fryer basket in it, grease it with cooking oil, shut the air fryer with its lid, set the temperature to 425 degrees F, and let it preheat.
- Meanwhile, prepare the peppers and for this, take a medium bowl, place rice in it, add tomatoes, oregano, salt, and onion powder and then stir until combined.
- Stuff the peppers with the rice mixture, arrange them in the air fryer in a single layer, spray oil on top, shut with its lid, and then cook for 10 to 15 minutes until done.
- Sprinkle 1 tablespoon cheese on top of the stuffed bell peppers, continue cooking for 5 minutes and then serve.

16. WILD RICE WITH CHICKPEAS AND MUSHROOMS

SERVING: 2

Preparation time: 5 minutes; Cook time: 12 minutes;
Nutritional Info: 161.5 Cal; 3.6 g Fats; 3.7 g Protein; 29.7 g Carb; 3 g Fiber;

INGREDIENTS

- 2 cups cooked wild rice
- ½ cup cooked chickpeas
- ¼ cup chopped mushrooms
- ½ of key lime, juiced
- 1 teaspoon sesame seeds oil

Extra:
- 1 teaspoon sea salt
- ½ teaspoon cayenne pepper

DIRECTIONS

- Plug in an air fryer, place the fryer basket in it, insert a baking pan in it greased with oil, shut the air fryer with its lid, set the temperature to 350 degrees F, and let it preheat.
- Meanwhile, take a large bowl, place rice in it, add mushrooms and chickpeas, stir in salt, cayenne pepper, lime juice, and oil, and stir until combined.
- Add the prepared rice mixture to the air fryer, shut with its lid, and then cook for 12 minutes until done, tossing frequently.
- Serve straight away.

17. WILD RICE WITH BELL PEPPERS AND TURNIP GREENS

SERVING: 2

Preparation time: 5 minutes; Cook time: 12 minutes;
Nutritional Info: 89.6 Cal; 2 g Fats; 2 g Protein; 17 g Carb; 2 g Fiber;

INGREDIENTS

- 2 cups cooked wild rice
- ½ cup cooked chickpeas
- ¼ cup bell pepper, chopped
- ½ cup turnip greens, chopped
- 1 teaspoon sesame seeds oil
- ½ of key lime, juiced
- 1 teaspoon sea salt
- ½ teaspoon cayenne pepper

DIRECTIONS

- Plug in an air fryer, place the fryer basket in it, insert a baking pan in it greased with oil, shut the air fryer with its lid, set the temperature to 350 degrees F, and let it preheat.
- Meanwhile, take a large bowl, place rice in it, add bell pepper and chickpeas, stir in salt, cayenne pepper, lime juice, and oil, and stir until combined.

- Add the prepared rice mixture to the air fryer, shut with its lid, and then cook for 10 minutes until done, tossing frequently.
- Add turnip greens into the air fryer, toss until mixed, and then continue cooking for 2 minutes.
- Serve straight away.

18. WILD RICE AND TOMATO LETTUCE WRAP

SERVING: 2

Preparation time: 5 minutes; Cook time: 10 minutes;
Nutritional Info: 147 Cal; 3 g Fats; 0 g Protein; 27 g Carb; 2 g Fiber;

INGREDIENTS

- 1 cup cooked wild rice
- 3 cherry tomatoes, chopped
- 1 tablespoon key lime juice
- 2 large lettuce leaves
- 1 teaspoon sesame seed oil
- ¼ teaspoon cayenne pepper
- ½ teaspoon sea salt

DIRECTIONS

- Plug in an air fryer, place the fryer basket in it, grease it with cooking oil, shut the air fryer with its lid, set the temperature to 250 degrees F, and let it preheat.
- Meanwhile, take a medium bowl, place rice in it, add tomatoes, salt, cayenne pepper, and key lime juice and then stir until combined.
- Add the rice mixture in the air fryer, spray oil on top, shut with its lid, and then cook for 5 minutes until thoroughly hot, turning halfway.
- Divide the rice mixture evenly between the lettuce leaves, wrap them and then serve.

19. BELL PEPPER STUFFED TEF

SERVING: 2

Preparation time: 5 minutes; Cook time: 20 minutes;
Nutritional Info: 45 Cal; 2 g Fats; 0.5 g Protein; 6 g Carb; 2 g Fiber;

INGREDIENTS

- 2 medium red bell peppers, cored

- 2 cherry tomatoes, chopped
- 1 cup cooked teff
- ½ teaspoon dried thyme
- 2 tablespoons hazel nut cheese
- ½ teaspoon cayenne pepper
- ½ teaspoon salt

DIRECTIONS

- Plug in an air fryer, place the fryer basket in it, grease it with cooking oil, shut the air fryer with its lid, set the temperature to 425 degrees F, and let it preheat.
- Meanwhile, prepare the peppers and for this, take a medium bowl, place teff in it, add tomatoes, thyme, salt, and cayenne pepper and then stir until combined.
- Stuff the peppers with the teff mixture, arrange them in the air fryer in a single layer, spray oil on top, shut with its lid, and then cook for 10 to 15 minutes until done.
- Sprinkle 1 tablespoon cheese on top of the stuffed bell peppers, continue cooking for 5 minutes and then serve.

RELATED BOOK YOU MAY LIKE

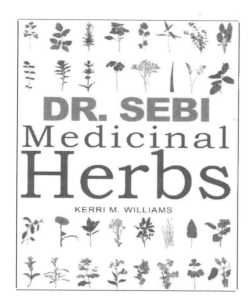

Dr. Sebi Medicinal Herbs

Healing Uses, Dosage, DIY Capsules & Where to buy wildcrafted Herbal Plants for Remedies, Detox Cleanse, Immunity, Weight loss, Body, Skin & Hair Rejuvenation

In the world we live in today, chronic diseases are on the rise, effectively making both conventional and alternative medicine a huge industry. And just when you realize that Americans spend more than $250 billion each year on drugs and supplements, then it's easier to understand how much of a problem the chronic disease pandemic has become. It's only human to want the best and safest, so we are naturally attracted to choose the most effective remedy – and worry about the side effects later. Be it food, drugs, herbs or supplement, we simply want the best – for health and healing. But the fact that what we see or hope to get isn't the reality is worrisome. Asides the effects of synthetic drugs and pills, many Americans often go with supplements because they believe it is healthier, costs less, has little side effects and most importantly, is "vital".

However, recent prescription drug recalls, have left much to be desired. Zantac, a popular H2 receptor blocker that treats severe cases of acid reflux and heartburn, was recently pulled off the shelf. Zantac was linked to Stomach cancer and many other drugs with similar mechanism of action were also implicated. Other drugs such as Accutane and Vioxx were not spared – in fact Vioxx in particular resulted in nearly 30,000 deaths and was used by more than 20 million people in a little over a 4-year span. These recalls and many others have further cast a doubt on not just conventional medicine, but the regulatory agencies including the U.S. Food and Drug Administration (FDA). But when you realize that the majority of Americans perceive the FDA's approval of drugs and food as a guarantee of safety and that all approval is based on "high degrees of clarity and certainty about a drug's risks and benefits", then you realize we may have a much bigger problem than we ever imagined.

When we look at all these, it begs the pertinent question – Can we really trust the conventional medical industry to seeking true holistic health and healing? Can we continue to put our health on the line for silly errors or slippages? How long can we continue to swallow every pill and hope ……

Made in the USA
Middletown, DE
29 June 2022